Palgrave Texts in Counselling and Psychotherapy

AF173572

Series Editors

Arlene Vetere
Family Therapy and Systemic Practice
VID Specialized University
Oslo, Norway

Rudi Dallos
Clinical Psychology
Plymouth University
Plymouth, UK

This series introduces readers to the theory and practice of counselling and psychotherapy across a wide range of topical issues. Ideal for both trainees and practitioners, the books will appeal to anyone wishing to use counselling and psychotherapeutic skills and will be particularly relevant to workers in health, education, social work and related settings. The books in this series emphasise an integrative orientation weaving together a variety of models including, psychodynamic, attachment, trauma, narrative and systemic ideas. The books are written in an accessible and readable style with a focus on practice. Each text offers theoretical background and guidance for practice, with creative use of clinical examples.

Arlene Vetere, Professor of Family Therapy and Systemic Practice at VID Specialized University, Oslo, Norway.

Rudi Dallos, Emeritus Professor, Dept. of Clinical Psychology, University of Plymouth, UK.

Tone Grover • Siv Merete Myra
Ulf Axberg
Editors

New Horizons in Systemic Practice with Adults

palgrave
macmillan

Editors
Tone Grover
Department of Family Therapy and
Systemic Practice
Faculty of Social Studies
VID Specialized University
Oslo, Norway

Siv Merete Myra
Department of Family Therapy and
Systemic Practice
Faculty of Social Studies
VID Specialized University
Oslo, Norway

Ulf Axberg
Department of Family Therapy and
Systemic Practice
Faculty of Social Studies
VID Specialized University
Oslo, Norway

ISSN 2662-9127   ISSN 2662-9135   (electronic)
Palgrave Texts in Counselling and Psychotherapy
ISBN 978-3-031-30525-2   ISBN 978-3-031-30526-9   (eBook)
https://doi.org/10.1007/978-3-031-30526-9

Cover illustration © Sergey Ryumin / Getty Images

This Palgrave Macmillan imprint is published by the registered company Springer Nature Switzerland AG.
The registered company address is: Gewerbestrasse 11, 6330 Cham, Switzerland

Acknowledgements

Behind a book there is always a great *we*. This book is no exception. Thanks to a wide range of contributors, we were able to start and finish this work. First and foremost, we want to give our deepest thanks to Jim Sheehan and Arlene Vetere. For years they have been an enormous inspiration and have made many contributions to our systemic family therapist milieu at VID Specialized University. They have also helped us connect with other systemic milieus as well as publishers in Europe. Quite simply, this book wouldn't have come into existence at all if it wasn't for them and their overwhelming generosity in guiding us.

We want also to express our gratitude to all our collaboration partners who seek to relate to their own lives, together with us, in what we call therapy rooms. Their living presence shows up, anonymized, in different parts of the chapters in this book. From them we have learned more than is possible to learn from any book. Without the inspiration received from them, this book would be empty in both a real and a metaphorical sense. As readers will see, rich contributions were received from all who supported this work by allowing themselves to be interviewed and by sharing their own time and insights with the authors.

We also want to thank VID Specialized University in Oslo, especially our Head of Studies Halvor de Flon and Dean Mona-Iren Hauge, for giving us the space, support and time needed to complete this work. The editors also owe a great debt to our professional "godfathers", Per Jensen and Håkon Hårtveit, who established our systemic family therapy education in Oslo. Thanks to their pioneering work, it has grown from a few enthusiastic people walking around in slippers to one of Europe's largest systemic training programs.

Last but not least our gratitude goes to our friends, families, partners and pets! They are there, for inspiration and insight, reminding us, every day, about how dependent we are on each other and giving inspiration to go deeper into the complexity and beauty of systemic understanding.

One final acknowledgement of dependence: all that is written here in this book by editors and authors rests on the shoulders of our wonderful colleagues, past and present, both from systemic milieus and from other disciplines. In systemic spirit, we don't want to make division between disciplines, and this richness is one of the reasons why we are so grateful to be part of systemic understanding.

With love,

Tone Grøver, Siv Merete Myra and Ulf Axberg

Contents

Notes on Contributors

Sigurd Riste Andersen is an assistant professor at VID Specialized University, Oslo, a position in which he teaches and supervises students in the areas of social work, child protection and family therapy and systemic practice. Being a passionate advocate of training and education, he is also the Managing Director of the University student clinic for family therapy. Sigurd has work experience with drug-related social work, family work in psychiatry and child welfare and with members of the refugee community. He is a board member of the Norwegian Family Therapy Association, has his own private practice as a couples and family therapist in Oslo and is engaged in preventive and health-promoting courses and projects. In his research, he is interested in education, supervision, clinical practice and therapy and existential themes.

Jennifer Aramini is a clinical psychologist. Her private practice deals with people who cope with depression, anxiety, substance abuse and eating disorders. She is vice-president of COMITES-Italian Association in Norway.

Ulf Axberg, PhD is Professor of Family Therapy and Systemic Practice at the VID Specialized University in Oslo, Norway. In addition, he is a licensed psychologist and psychotherapist and clinical supervisor. He has long experience working in Child and Adolescent Mental Health and Social Services. His main research interests are systemic intervention, parental support and children exposed to intimate partner violence. He has authored and co-authored several articles in peer-reviewed journals and book chapter.

Bård Bertelsen is an associate professor at the University of Agder, in Kristiansand and Grimstad, where he is a manager of the Psychology Academic Group and teacher and supervisor for students in family therapy and psychosocial health. He is also a clinical psychologist specializing in family psychology and child and youth psychology. In his research, he has been interested in parenthood in post-divorce conflict and the social organization of family therapy and other psychotherapy practices.

Nicoletta Businaro is Associate Professor of Family Therapy and Systemic Practice at VID Specialized University, Oslo. She holds a PhD and Postdoc in psychology and has a specialization as a family therapist. Her research, didactic and practice interests are related to systemic family therapy, developmental psychology and the approach of positive psychology. She is author and co-author of several international articles and book chapters that regard cultural aspects involved in therapeutic process, disability, children's subjective well-being and emotional development.

Tone Grøver is an associate professor at VID Specialized University, Oslo, is a sociologist, has a master's degree in systemic family therapy and has a specialist education in narrative psychotherapy. She has worked for over 20 years as a private therapist for couples, families and individuals. She has also worked on assignments for the public and private sectors with conflicts, work environment challenges and conversations with managers (coaching) for almost 30 years. She has published three works of fiction and in her teaching she emphasizes a narrative form. She is interested in the insights we gain in therapy through art and poetic language.

Åse Holmberg, PhD is an ssociate professor of family therapy and systemic practice at VID Specialized University in Oslo, working with teaching, research and supervision. Her PhD from 2018 explored what spirituality means for family therapeutic practice, and she continues to work with spirituality and existential perspectives in various systemic contexts. She has also been a private family therapist for over 20 years, for couples, families and individuals.

Bengt Karlsson works at the University of South-Eastern Norway at the Faculty of Health and Social Sciences, Institute of Health, Social and Welfare Studies. Bengt holds a professorship in mental health care and is the leader of Centre for Mental Health and Substance Abuse. He trained as psychiatric nurse as well as a family therapist. His main areas of research are within recovery, collaborative research, open dialogue and human rights.

Siv Merete Myra is an associate professor at VID Specialized University, Oslo, Norway, since 2014. She completed her postgraduate dissertation in 2018 with the University of Oslo, Faculty of Medicine. She is a member of the Faculty of Social Studies at VID Specialized University where she teaches family therapy to master's-level students. She has been working in specialized health care for 25 years with families and children in the addiction field. She supervises therapists in the field of addiction, child welfare and family therapy. Her primary systemic practice interest is children and families living with substance abuse disorder and the prevention of intergenerational transference. Her research has been related to substance-abusing pregnant women in compulsory and voluntary treatment settings in Norway and their therapists.

Anne Øfsti is an associate professor at VID Specialized University, Oslo, Norway, where she is responsible for the professional training of couple and family therapists. Her doctoral thesis is entitled *Some Call It Love: Exploring Norwegian Therapists Discourses About Love and Intimacy.* She has presented her work in Norway and in other countries and has also published in peer-reviewed journals. Previously she was the editor for the Scandinavian journal *Fokus på familien* (Systemic Practice and Family Therapy). She has extensive professional experience as a couple and family therapist and supervisor. In 2014, she debuted as a novelist, with the title *If Only We Had All Day* which is a story about shame, guilt, forgiveness and hope, and of course family relations.

Leandra Perrotta, PsyD is an Italo-Australian clinical psychologist and specialist in psychotherapy. Leandra is a teacher, supervisor and co-founder of the Anne Ancelin Schützenberger International School of Transgenerational Therapy, and a teacher at IPAP—Post Graduate Institute of Analytical Psychology and Jungian Psychotherapy. She is former President of FEPTO—Federation of European Psychodrama Training Organizations—and a member of the FEPTO Task Force for Peace Building and Conflict Transformation. She has a fondness for literature and holds a master's degree in English and French Literature. Leandra has held lectures, workshops and trainings in psychodrama, dance movement therapy, transgenerational therapy, trauma, dreams and sexuality in over 40 different countries worldwide. Leandra has authored and co-authored 20 international articles and book chapters.

Jim Sheehan is Professor Emeritus of Family Therapy and Systemic Practice at VID Specialized University, Oslo. He is a systemic family therapist, trainer and systemic supervisor with a background of more than 30 years of practice as a social worker. He lives and practices in the Republic of Ireland. His recent publications include *Family Conflict After Separation and Divorce* (2018, Palgrave) and two edited texts with Arlene Vetere: *Long Term Systemic Therapy* (2020, Palgrave) and *Supervision of Family Therapy and Systemic Practice* (2017, Springer).

Inger-Margrete Svendsen is a specialist psychologist who has worked as a researcher at the Work Research Institute and has had her private practice as clinical psychologist and therapist for adults since 1996. She is a supervisor for psychologists, as well as for different teams and groups in the public and private sector. She has broad experience in working with conflicts in work life and in families. She is passionately engaged with the topic of conversations in human lives, and much of her work revolves around the importance of building trust in relationships.

Thomas Bernhard Thiis-Evensen has a Cand. Philos.-degree in History of Ideas from the University of Oslo, working as a philosophical practitioner (NSFP) at Diakonhjemmet Omsorg AS. He is a board member of the Educational Committee of the Norwegian Society of Philosophical Practice (NSFP), teaching and supervising students. He works mainly with existential themes, existential health, and quality of life through philosophically oriented communities of inquiry both one on one and with groups of people in vulnerable life circumstances (long-term survivors of HIV/AIDS [Pioneers], seniors, addicts and next of kin, persons breaking with religion, persons living with amyotrophic lateral sclerosis

[ALS], etc.). Through funded projects using systematic user feedback, he has developed methods and courses for volunteers and people working with people wanting to work more existentially informed.

Arlene Vetere is Professor Emeritus of Family Therapy and Systemic Practice at VID Specialized University, Oslo. She is a clinical psychologist and systemic psychotherapist, trainer and supervisor, registered in the UK, where she resides. She has recently edited two texts with Jim Sheehan: *Long Term Systemic Therapy* (2020, Palgrave) and *Supervision of Family Therapy and Systemic Practice* (2017, Springer).

1

Editors' Introduction

Tone Grover, Siv Merete Myra, and Ulf Axberg

This book will introduce you, the reader, to the reasons why systemic theory, as a meta-theory and a relational organic theory, is a suitable framework for understanding and appreciating the new horizons of therapeutic practice that are described in the chapters that follow. This book is written in times of uncertainty at many levels. So, more than ever, we experience how dependent we all are on each other and that this dependence seems to have no limits.

Systemic thinking is a way of understanding our being in the world, from the big questions to the small choices we make together. Therapy and therapeutic processes are also part of our being in the world together. We want this book to shed light on these processes and explore how we can develop systemic therapy and systemic understanding, from the small micro-choices we make towards each other to opening up the larger questions about what therapy can be, and how we should understand the ethics of what we do in the light of our times.

T. Grover (✉) • S. M. Myra • U. Axberg
Department of Family Therapy and Systemic Practice, Faculty of Social Studies, VID Specialized University, Oslo, Norway
e-mail: tone.grover@vid.no

© The Author(s), under exclusive license to Springer Nature Switzerland AG 2023
T. Grover et al. (eds.), *New Horizons in Systemic Practice with Adults*, Palgrave Texts in Counselling and Psychotherapy, https://doi.org/10.1007/978-3-031-30526-9_1

The different chapters will explore how systemic perspectives, as they are presented in the various practice contexts of the authors, can promote hope by giving room for reflections on uncertainty, change, opportunities, interconnections and differences. Furthermore, the chapters will illuminate the ways that systemic theory makes space for a multiplicity of varying approaches that address the needs of all of us in the different settings where we live our lives, and maybe seek therapy.

So why do we need this book about new horizons for systemic practice with adults and families? We wanted to explore newer applications of understanding and development in systemic practice and show how a growing integration of current research with these new developments across the broader fields of psychotherapy and counselling can be held within a systemic relational umbrella. In this book, we focus on existential themes and on how insights from the different realms of science, literature and history, as well as learning from our clients and our nurturing communities, can be included within a systemic understanding that embraces different therapeutic perspectives.

The emphasis in this book is on the social utility of the approaches and perspectives presented, their historical origins and how practice can be enhanced as a result. All of the editors and authors are leading some of the developments in their particular field of competence. Several of the authors are affiliated with VID Specialized University, Oslo, while others are systemic practitioners and trainers from other parts of Norway and Europe. All the authors use examples from their systemic practice across a range of contexts and themes. Each chapter will explore aspects of working with difference and diversity as a golden thread and orient the reader to new practices in changing and changed working contexts. Themes of loneliness and separation, marginalisation and exclusion, safety and protection, play and exploration, evil and forgiveness, health and death, spirituality and healing, and trust in its many subtle forms have always been with us, but in a time of uncertainty, our awareness of how such existential issues impact in our daily lives has intensified. This book is written with love for the depth of systemic understanding, for its complexity, and not least for its ability to realise how dependent we all are on each other. Each chapter will translate some of these themes directly into practice examples, learning points and tips for practitioners.

Chapter 2 (Jim Sheehan and Arlene Vetere) introduces us to a Systemic View of Agape in therapy. The chapter starts like this: "Love. Straight to the heart of therapy. So why do we talk and write about alliances, therapeutic relationships, goals, tasks and bonds? Do we risk hiding behind our research-based descriptors? Are they a form of institutional defence that is protective for both of us as practitioners and our clients—a fear of unhelpful boundary crossing perhaps? Fears of dual relationships, sexual exploitation, or countertherapeutic practice? Is this why we do not call our therapeutic relationships love?" Enjoy this chapter—as Tina Turner's sang: What's love got to do with it?

Chapter 3 (Tone Grøver and Inger-Margrete Svendsen) is written as a letter to you as the reader. The authors invite you to explore your own experiences with trust in therapy. From systemic theory, we know a lot about what creates trust. However, this is mostly at a somewhat general level, such as the meaning of listening, accepting, respecting and representing equality. The authors wish to be specific, looking at micro-situations and the subtleties of little sequences, where much of our experience lies and our lives are shaped and ask: What is it that gives rise to trust? What are the forms of expression of trust? All the way through the chapter they ask questions to you, the reader. And they invite you to send them a letter about your experiences so that a continuation of this exploration could be made by you and your collaboration partners.

Chapter 4 (Anne Øfsti and Bård Bertelsen) questions forgiveness. The chapter takes its place within a long and rich tradition of systemic thinking on forgiveness. The authors suggest that they find, both in their personal lives and their practice, a strong expectation that we should forgive. This prevailing discourse is challenged through an interweaving of stories from personal life and practice experience. Like other systemic thinkers before them (Sheehan, 2007), they have turned towards philosophers like Arendt and Derrida to throw further light on the many paradoxes generated by the theme as it presents both in personal life and in practice.

Chapter 5 (Tone Grøver) is about longing and the longing for oneself. It is often expressed with this sentence "I have lost myself." The chapter discusses whether the premise that we are separate selves has come to be valid in systemic therapy and therefore whether we have inadvertently abandoned what might be a key point in systemic understanding. The chapter discusses the consequences of therapy if we were to assume that the separate self is a fundamentally false premise in the sciences of people and society. The author also asks if the premise of the separate self, and longing, might play an important part in our ongoing destruction of the earth.

Chapter 6 (Åse Holmberg and Bengt Karlsson) is about giving resonance and room to spirituality in systemic practice. The chapter explores the concept of spirituality underpinned by voices from an ongoing study of unemployed young adults in Norway. The authors link spirituality to systemic perspectives, like love, wondering and complexity. Finally, they encourage systemic family therapists to find their own spiritual path which in turn can perhaps make us more open to our clients' spiritual lives.

Chapter 7 (Anne Øfsti) explores how literary fiction can move, touch and create insights into what it is to live, individually and together, in different ways than traditional scientific literature can. The author says: "I dare to claim that reading and writing fiction has shaped me as a therapist in completely different ways than non-fiction and research texts. I think it is a loss that fiction has less knowledge status than the evidence-based research texts." The chapter offers us a description of a reading group in a systemic therapist training programme, couched in the author's love of literature.

Chapter 8 (Sigurd Riste and Thomas Bernhard Thiis-Evensen) is an exploration of existential themes in couples therapy from the perspective of therapists. In this chapter, the authors explore their own wonderings and show, with an example, how we might explore such phenomena as identity, meaning, sickness and death, freedom, responsibility, choice, remorse, guilt, shame, loneliness, relations and attachment *in an existential way*.

Chapter 9 (Nicoletta Businaro, Leandra Perrotta and Jennifer Aramini) has the title "Should I stay, or Should I Go? Rethinking Identity and the Experience of Migration as a Systemic Dialogue in Therapy." The chapter focuses on a topic that is relatively unexplored in the family therapy literature: what happens in the therapy room when therapist and client have experienced migration, and both have the same country of origin.

The authors illustrate some resources and possible traps in this specific context using some clinical vignettes.

Chapter 10 (Sigurd Riste) invites therapists into the question: What if we only met once? The chapter is inspired by Single Session Therapy, but it is not a description of SST; rather, it takes inspiration from the deeply creative work that can occur if we do not plan for more than one meeting.

Chapter 11 (Arlene Vetere) explores the part neuroscience can play in a re-understanding of therapy. With the benefit of observation and feedback over years of experience, psychotherapists have always known how to intuitively respond to their clients' states of mind and physiological readiness to address their particular difficulties. It is this attuned awareness of what constitutes relational safety and relational danger, for all of us, that is one hallmark of systemic practice. Now, with the advent of polyvagal theory, and advances in modern attachment theory, we are in a position to understand better the neurological mechanisms underpinning emotional experience, and the regulation and co-regulation of arousal. We can ask what the central nervous system needs in the face of relational dangers.

In our Epilogue, the editors reflect on some of the many questions posed by the authors in their chapters. Far from making conclusions of any kind, we invite you, our readers, into further reflections of your own on what we perceive as the new horizons emerging in our systemic field. We do this in a spirit of connection not just between authors, editors and readers in the present but also between all of us in the present and all those known and less-known persons from the past who built and rebuilt the tradition of systemic therapy without which we could not envision new horizons shaping the present and future.

You're so welcome!

Reference

Sheehan, J. (2007). Forgiveness and the unforgivable: The resurrection of hope in family therapy. In *Hope and despair in narrative and family therapy*. Routledge.

2

The Therapeutic Relationship: A Systemic View of Agape

Jim Sheehan and Arlene Vetere

Love. Straight to the heart of therapy. So why do we talk and write about alliances, therapeutic relationships, goals, tasks, and bonds? Do we risk hiding behind our research-based descriptors? Are they a form of institutional defence that is protective for both of us as practitioners and our clients—a fear of unhelpful boundary crossing perhaps? Fears of dual relationships, sexual exploitation, or countertherapeutic practice? Is this why we do not call our therapeutic relationships love? In our therapeutic work, we have the capacity to make and sustain deeply felt and committed connections, grounded in interpersonal trust and infused with compassion, care, and empathy. We could say these are the vital ingredients in a loving relationship—that therapy is an experience of mutual love and loving. So perhaps the apparently one-sided nature of the therapeutic relationship, with formal responsibility for the therapy resting with the practitioner, challenges our ideas of mutual interest and reciprocity in love. However, there is reciprocity in therapy, with different roles, responsibilities, relational esteem, and mutual learning, but nonetheless, a

J. Sheehan (✉) • A. Vetere
VID Specialized University, Oslo, Norway

profound exchange and an immersion in the life of another or others. As Martin Buber wrote: 'To step into elemental relation with the other … requires and creates the most intensive stirring of one's being' (1988, p. 71).

So, this chapter is about love, love at the centre and heart of the therapeutic relationship. It is about remembering something we already know about our work but have somehow forgotten. It is about acknowledging something prior to all practice methodologies and formats, prior to therapeutic alliances, and prior to all practice protocols, goals, and tasks. It is about a love that gives rise to the therapeutic relationship, continues to fuel its functioning and development, and is the ongoing source of its many fruits. It is about a kind of love that is most accurately described as *agape*. But what kind of love is agape? How can we detect its presence in therapeutic work, and how does it function therein? Can and should agape have a clear voice of its own within the therapeutic relationship or should it make its presence felt through specific behaviours and actions of the relationship participants? These are some of the questions that have informed the reflections the reader will find in this chapter. The chapter will begin with a brief overview of some different meanings that have surrounded the concept of agape love in general as well as the meanings it has acquired in its use in the specific context of therapeutic work performed through different therapeutic modalities. This overview is a prelude to our holding side by side the concept of agape love and a range of sensitivities that have emerged over several decades in systemic theory and practice, sensitivities that have alluded to love without always naming love. Indeed, with the possible exception of Satir (1988), there has been a general reluctance within the major systemic theorists over the last half-century to name the presence of love in therapy and the therapeutic relationship. We will consider some possible sources of this reluctance on the way to articulating a specifically systemic view of agape.

If this chapter is about acknowledging the significance of love at the heart of the therapeutic and associated relationships such as the supervisory relationship, it is equally about the risks encountered by clients, professionals, and agencies when love and its demands are forgotten, ignored, sidelined, or suppressed. It is our belief that there are many aspects of the contemporary culture surrounding therapeutic practice in health, social care, and private practice settings that contribute to this forgetfulness and suppression. When the culture of science so envelopes the field of therapy that its functioning as art is eclipsed, we concomitantly sideline the art of loving that is at the heart of its constitution and forget that our therapeutic practices have a shared foothold in science and art, a foothold that we consider mutually informing. When the culture of legislative frameworks and mandatory protocols governing practice takes centre stage and preoccupies service managers and their managed therapists, therapeutic practice runs the risk of becoming fear-based and defensive. In the process, this culture can unwittingly foster the alienation of clients from their treatment, therapists from their therapeutic art, and agencies from their mission. Finally, in identifying the risks to love, we respond by exploring some possible protective and promotional measures proportionate to the phenomenon of agape as it can be felt, experienced, and enjoyed by systemic therapists, their clients, and systemic supervisors. While we acknowledge the presence of agape in all therapeutic relationships, we think it is particularly noticeable for practitioners, clients, and supervisees in the context of longer-term therapeutic and supervisory relationships.

How We Came to Write This Chapter

What is it in our respective experiences that have moved us to write this chapter together on love at the heart of therapy? As the years went by, I, Arlene, found myself increasingly feeling that what was happening in therapy, and what I was experiencing, was love. A form of love that gladly gives of itself and seeks nothing more. In the words of Kahlil Gibran, 'Work is love made visible' (1923). For me, Jim, it was the experience of a deeply felt joy arising and growing in me in the context of many different therapeutic relationships. A joy for which I could find no other explanation than the mutual love and loving at the heart of each unique therapeutic relationship, each oriented towards its own unique set of goals. In each of these relationships, I came to see that I was immersed in an ever-evolving circle of love and joy. If these are some of the more personal roots of our journeys towards loving love, we turn now to some of the historical roots of the agape concept within our cultures and therapeutic traditions.

The Conceptual Belonging of Agape

The term *agape* first appeared in the Hellenistic Greek translation of the Old Testament and was used even more widely in the New Testament (Lambert, 1973). Within the Old Testament translation, the term agape was used to depict a wide range of love contexts such as family love, the love of Samson for Delilah, the love of Hosea for his adulterous wife, as well as the love of God for human beings and vice versa. Some commentators (Sanday & Headam, 1908) have noted that this broad range of meanings for the concept did not exclude other meanings such as severity, anger, and hatred. While this breadth of meaning was maintained in the New Testament, the concept only later became transformed in some Christian cultures into a rather sharp distinction between *eros* and *agape*. While the former came to depict sexualized, passionate forms of love, the latter idea referred to 'a rather more spiritualized non-erotic care for the eternal destiny of others arising from the action of God upon the soul and not from the feelings and emotions of human beings' (Lambert, 1973). One of the most often-quoted texts on love within the more recent Christian tradition is St Paul's First Epistle to the Corinthians (Chapter 13, verses 4–8) which commences 'Love is always patient and kind; love is never jealous etc.' Such a perspective on agape, Lambert (1973) notes, is an idealized view of love which fails to give a legitimate place in the human psyche and relationships to the challenging emotions of hatred, envy, jealousy, pride, and so on, what Jungians might call the shadow side. In a systemic perspective on agape within the therapeutic relationship, we want to retain some of the breadth of the earlier meanings which we think imply two things: firstly, they acknowledge the potential presence of many difficult emotions and experiences within and between therapists and clients and the integration and containment of these over time in ways that free individuals for new ways of relating to, and loving, both self and others; and secondly, they point to the presence within the therapist from the outset of a willingness to be as fully present to and for the client(s) as possible, of a caring, patient, and kindly disposition, and a preparedness to maintain an unconditional positive regard (Rogers, 1992) for the client/others.

A systemic view of agape, we suggest, acknowledges the presence of love in the therapeutic relationship from the beginning. It perceives agape as the source of the impulse which prompts our 'yes' to the invitation to become involved in the lives of the traumatized and wounded, as the energy which sustains therapists and clients on the sometimes very long journey towards integrating seemingly impossible experiences, and as the light which gives hope to the next part of the journey for both clients and therapists. Indeed, the work undertaken within and through the therapeutic relationship is a labour of love from start to finish, despite this love having different textures at different points along the way. While we recognize that many cultures in the world endorse perspectives on agape which carry divine or transcendent meanings as their centre point, these are not the perspectives we are advancing in this chapter. The systemic perspective on agape described here is a fully human agape which has its roots in the neurobiology of human beings (the neurobiologists tell us that we are literally wired for love) and is a love which grows and develops in their attachment bonds and relationships. It is a love that is nurtured and deepened through the patient, reflexive, reception and examination of the lived and told stories of both clients and therapists and is immanent within their evolving relationship.

While the systemic tradition may have been particularly silent on the theme of love within the therapeutic relationship, this has not been the case in some other psychotherapy modalities. Snyder (2000) reminds us that, notwithstanding their different ways of describing the phenomenon of love and its functioning, therapists from most therapeutic traditions have felt that it makes sense to love one's clients and experience the mutuality of that love. We will confine ourselves here to looking at a small group of perspectives and themes relating to love coming from the psychoanalytic tradition. We consider it unsurprising that some of the most interesting reflections on love within the therapeutic relationship have come from that part of the psychotherapy 'family' most noted for long-term engagement with clients and for the long-term supervision of psychoanalysts in training and practice.

'Therapeutic Love' Within the Psychoanalytic Tradition

The idea of love within the analytic relationship has a rich and interesting history within psychoanalysis. As a concept, it was greatly debated and contested between two of the tradition's founders, Sigmund Freud and his one-time student and later colleague, Sandor Ferenczi. Many of the abiding questions about the nature of therapeutic love shared between therapists and clients have their origins in this debate. While their positions shared a great deal in the beginning, differences between them on the topic grew over time and eventually Freud's theory of *libido* would overshadow Ferenczi's focus on *love* for several decades. It will be of interest to systemic practitioners that Freud's early work was imbued with a great deal more relationality than is revealed in his later work on the science of drives. In that earlier phase, the progress of the patient/analysand depended, for Freud, on the continuing respect and sympathy of the doctor/analyst for the patient. In 1906, Freud wrote in his fourth letter to Jung: 'Essentially, one might say, the cure is effected by love … and transference' (Freud/Jung Letters, pp. 2–13). In this communication, transference, we are told by Lothane (1996), should not be seen as referring to the satisfaction of the patient's real sexual demands, but in fact 'pointed to love writ large, to that fire within, the ardent and passionate emotions that make life worth living' (Lothane, 1996, p. 216). In the same letter to Jung, he underscored the emotional power of transference, a term he later reaffirmed as a synonym for love (Lothane, 1998).

However, when Freud later made the libido of the sexual instincts the centre of his emerging science of psychoanalysis, all other phenomena that might appear in the analytic relationship such as the nonsexual love of *agape* or the 'liking' love of *philia* became derivatives of the sexual drive. It was this upturning of the place of love within the analytic relationship that saw the commencement of the rift between master and student. Unlike Freud, Ferenczi generated and retained a dyadic/relational understanding of real childhood traumas such as child sexual abuse that became the basis of later adult neurosis and other symptomatology. For

Ferenczi, love was the critical component of the analysis, the factor without which the treatment could not be effective (Ferenczi, 1932).

However, it was on the ground of *expressions* of love for the patient that Freud had most disagreement with Ferenczi. There appears to have been a brief period within the latter's practice when he used to kiss some of his patients. As this became public knowledge within the psychoanalytic community, Freud was swift in his admonition of his ex-student and was unequivocal in his view that physical intimacy has no place within the psychoanalytic relationship. The psychotherapy tradition owes a debt of gratitude to these figures for kick-starting a debate not only about the place of therapeutic love within the therapeutic relationship but also about the manner in which love should find legitimate expression therein.

A much more recent contribution to the debate about therapeutic love and its expression is made from within one of psychoanalysis's many derivative modalities, the domain of Functional Analytic Psychotherapy (Munoz-Martinez & Follette, 2019). While noting the difficulty the concept of love presents for researchers, these authors are equally concerned about the challenges presented by using the *love* word within the therapeutic relationship. They comment: 'Almost every client and therapist has a history of what the word love means. If that word gets introduced in therapy, it has whatever meaning the therapist intends plus unknown additional meaning based upon the history that each party has with the word and experiences paired with the word' (Munoz-Martinez & Follette, 2019, p. 105). For these authors, the concept of therapeutic love brings practitioners to the edge of critical ethical obligations. These obligations can be summed up in two maxims: first, that client goals should always be the guide for therapist behaviour in the session, so that therapeutic actions are only intended to benefit clients; and second, that ethical caring should always be the touchstone of therapeutic love behaviours (Tsai et al., 2013). While endorsing the importance of a loving environment within the therapeutic relationship and affirming that therapy is likely to be more effective when the therapist cares deeply for the well-being of the client, these authors express considerable concern about the use within the therapeutic relationship of what they term *I love you* and equivalent behaviours. We will return later in this chapter to consider in more detail what a systemic position on expressions of love within the therapeutic relationship might entail.

Indeed, it is likely that an enduring, and understandable, anxiety surrounding the risks of boundary transgression in the longer-term treatment of vulnerable adults has played an important role in a turning away from the theme of therapeutic love in most psychotherapeutic modalities. This 'turning away from love' within psychotherapy was, perhaps, further fostered by the increasing impetus towards putting therapeutic practices of all kinds on a secure scientific footing. There was something about the very theme of love that did not appear to sit well with the drive towards evidence-based practices within most psychotherapeutic modalities. One of the psychoanalytic voices from the past who refused to see any dichotomy between love and a rigorous scientific disposition and the objectivity it implies was that of Loewald (1980). Writing about the analytic relationship, Loewald wrote about the intertwining of love and science in the following way:

> Scientific detachment in its genuine form, far from excluding love, is based on it. In our work it can truly be said that in our best moments of dispassionate and objective analysis, we love our object, the patient, more than at any other time and are compassionate with his whole being. In our field scientific spirit and care for the object flow from the same source. (Loewald, 1980, p. 297)

Reflections on Agape Within the Systemic Tradition

While we have already noted that the systemic tradition has been relatively silent regarding explicit naming of therapeutic love, a silence we believe has been shared by many other psychotherapy modalities, there have been notable exceptions to this within the last two decades. In this section, we want to describe two of these contributions. The first of these is provided by Snyder (2000), who argues for the necessity of love being mutual in the therapeutic relationship if it is to be healing. The second is provided by Seikkula and Trimble (2005), who see the dialogical processes underpinning therapeutic conversations as 'an embodiment of love'.

For Snyder, love is the appropriate term to describe a significant therapeutic relationship 'in which there is mutual empathy and respect and to which the client can bring everything that he thinks and feels and be met by the therapist's authentic caring' (Snyder, 2000, p. 4). Snyder points initially to the work of Schafer who saw analytic love as being bound up with a quality of 'focused attentiveness' that moves the therapist beyond the limits of a theoretical model into the 'face-to-face'. She sees in Gergen's concept of 'the relational sublime' (Gergen, 1996) an indicator of those non-verbalizable ways of knowing that have been considered by many as central to the capacity to love. And she endorses Maturana and Varela's (1987) attribution of love to biological roots and their description of love's nature as 'the opening of space for the other to exist' (Snyder, 2000, p. 6). Central to Snyder's position, however, is the importance of exploring power differences (a theme to be explored more fully in a later section of this chapter) with respect to race, class, gender, education, sexuality, and so on if therapy is to be a truly relational event. And while systems of ethical rules and their enforcement are always necessary for the protection of clients and therapists, of much greater priority for her is 'the full consideration of particular human beings in their particular contexts' (Snyder, 2000, p. 7).

Snyder wonders why a focus on the risks (sexual acting out, the therapist's needs interfering with the therapy, cultivating an unnecessary relational interdependency) associated with therapeutic love have so often outweighed a focus on, and commitment to, mutual love within the therapeutic relationship even in the face of love's acknowledged importance. One reason she advances concerns the challenges raised for therapists when their clients respond to them with a fuller and more intense emotional engagement. This can evoke a fear of love in therapists who then deploy what Jordan et al. (1991) call 'strategies of disconnection' as means of protecting themselves from potential hurt. However, the therapeutic attunement of the therapist in these contexts of disconnection must move them towards a recognition of their own protective strategies and a willingness to address them with the client. The self-disclosure and therapist transparency that this requires often brings a mutuality of empathy, which Snyder considers an integral part of love and healing. For Snyder, change and transformation are possible for both client and therapist when the therapeutic relationship remains a loving relationship and when that love 'includes authenticity, vulnerability, and dialogic cocreation' (Snyder, 2000, p. 17).

Seikkula and Trimble (2005) do not focus directly on the theme of therapeutic love but recognize that feelings of love are emergent within the therapeutic processes attaching to the Open Dialogue (Seikkula et al., 1995) approach to the treatment of serious psychological conditions. This approach is characterized by two key elements: the organization of the treatment system and the dialogic process through which meetings are conducted. Regarding the first of these factors, what is critical is that the patient, their family network, and the professional team all meet together and no decisions about treatment are made outside of this network that continues to meet for as long as is necessary. The process does not depend on 'some brilliant intervention by the professional', but its effectiveness lies 'in the emotional exchange among network members, including the professionals, who together construct or restore a caring personal community' (Seikkula & Trimble, 2005, p. 462). The process moves slowly to allow for the different rhythms and styles of each network member to be incorporated in the meeting. The process proceeds through the support of a 'polyphonic' engagement between the voices of the client, their network, and the team.

Research investigations into the workings of this dialogic approach suggest that the critical factors in healing are the 'creation of new, shared language from multivoiced conversation, shared emotional experience, and creation of community, all of which...are supported by powerful mutual emotional attunement, an experience that most people would recognize as experiences of love' (Seikkula & Trimble, 2005, p. 465). Within the process, team members are encouraged to participate as fully embodied persons, aware of their own emotional responses resonating with other emotions in the room. Network members also learn that they can depend on the support of team members to assist them to remain engaged in conversation about difficult matters that they had been unable to contain in previous efforts between themselves. The authors comment that the feelings of love that emerge in team members during a network meeting 'are neither romantic nor erotic. They are our own embodied responses to participation in a shared world of meaning cocreated with people who trust each other and ourselves to be transparent, comprehensive beings with each other'.

As we write of these systemic windows on agapic love, we remind ourselves that *agape*, as a Greco-Christian concept, has also been defined as a form of unconditional love that transcends particular circumstances and persists through both chronological and subjective times. For example, Rogers' (1992) work on unconditional positive regard—empathy, genuineness, and warmth—is seen as a form of non-possessive love or agape. It is in the therapeutic process where the therapist affirms, values, and accepts the client/s that, in turn, family members have more opportunity to develop acceptance, self-love, and love for the others. This Rogerian perspective set the scene for the shorter-term psychotherapies to both establish and validate the connection between the practitioner and the client as the ongoing vehicle for change (Castonguay et al., 2006). Currently though, and sad to say, the trend for goals and target achievement in therapy can make it harder to hold on to Rogers' attitude and notions of love.

In the practice of systemic therapy, there are usually more than two people involved, and as the family is understood to be part of the solution to the problem, the therapist will often decentre themselves in the search for strengths and resilient responses. Then, with the advent of reflecting teams and processes (Andersen, 1992), and the use of training teams, more people became involved, and perhaps this somehow diluted the sense of intense or intimate connection and distributed (or even diluted?) the feeling of connection more as a collective responsibility and a shared fondness for the family members. For systemic therapists in training, their work is under scrutiny and evaluation from a number of perspectives, and any resultant felt anxiety may inhibit the focus on and the deepening of connections in favour of visible competence with interventions.

Most of the systemic writing on engagement and joining (e.g., Minuchin, 1974) focuses on the earlier stages of the development of the therapeutic relationship—we suggest here that it is not enough to make a good working relationship, it is important to know how to continue to develop it and use it in the service of the family members' relational development—thus may we explore the deeper recesses of experiences and heal disturbances of experiencing—'making the unknown known'.

As we can see from all of the above, there are many philosophies, theories, and languages of love. Love is complex—it interconnects with cultural views and traditions on parenting and marriage/partnership, forms of intimacy, affection, sex, power and control, life cycle, and emotions of joy, fear, sadness, and shame (Lago & Charura, 2016). There have been many attempts to capture the essence of the experience of love, and in doing so we risk losing sight of the whole experience—in systemic theory, the concept of 'the whole is greater than the sum of the parts' helps to illustrate this dilemma. In writing this chapter, we are focusing on love in therapy as agape—unconditional warmth, respect, mutual empathy, and regard as the basis for interpersonal trust and therapeutic growth in which family members' love experiences and perspectives interplay with those of the therapist.

Power and Difference

We have already noted the importance of the phenomena of power and difference within the systemic tradition. But how do we manage power differentials in a therapeutically loving relationship? And how do we manage these dimensions in a way that promotes an ongoing experience of safety for the therapy participants including the therapist? This is an acquired skill for practitioners, often based on past experience of caring roles, for family members, friends, animals, and significant others. Without this skill, supporting people who are currently vulnerable and dependent can be overwhelming, with the concomitant responses of either rigidity and rule following (dismissive tendencies) or the more chaotic difficulty with emotional boundary and arousal regulation (preoccupied strategies).

There has been an emphasis on the systemic therapies on use of self, relational reflexivity (or talking about talking), and the impact of social context on relationships and well-being. Burnham (2005) defines relational reflexivity as 'the intention, desire, processes and practices through which therapists and clients explicitly engage one another in coordinating their resources so as to create a relationship with therapeutic potential'. It is usual in therapeutic and supervisory practice to explore social and structural issues, such as age, ethnicity, gender, faith, class and sexuality, and their intersections in people's lives, including that of the therapist and supervisor. These explorations are not taken for granted; rather they are negotiated, discussed, and developed with an awareness of the use and misuse of power, in therapy, in supervision, and in life outside. In order to understand and be of assistance, we need to engage with this complexity; bear witness to experiences of disconnection, marginalization, and hurt; manage strong feelings and moral outrage at injustice; and support empowerment and healing. Snyder (2000) observes that when working therapeutically with experiences of both external and/or internal oppression, it may be necessary to give up privilege, power, or deeply held beliefs, and this may involve losses of different kinds. The therapist needs to pay attention to self-care with the help of supervision. When working with experiences of injustice and relational danger, we are trying, more often than not, to make new meanings where none seem to exist.

There are many aspects to creating a felt experience of safety in therapeutic work with couples and families. The therapist's responsibility and capacity to work in a responsive, open, and accessible way also interacts with family members' sense of safety with each other in the therapeutic work, their views of the therapeutic relationship, their therapist and the therapy goals, and their separate and shared willingness to experiment with change. The therapeutic relationship is itself layered systemically: each family member with the therapist, with each other, with their collective identity, and the therapist with the couple/family group. None of the foregoing suggests that there are not moments when safety in the therapeutic relationship is not seriously threatened, when the power and force of negative emotions such as hatred, resentment, and bitterness look like they will run the work into the ground. It is in these moments, which can sometimes extend over a number of sessions, that agape finds its greatest test. And the test is faced by the enduring presence and expression of the therapist's compassion for self and others. It is this multidirectional compassion that keeps the work steady and progressing in difficult conditions and offers the hope of emergence from what may be felt like therapeutic ordeal with new vision and capacity for all joined in the work, including the therapist. We cannot underline sufficiently the place of importance held by the supervisory relationship in the holding steady of the therapist's therapeutic work in these moments when agape is severely tested.

Therapy as an Attachment Process

A further window into love within the systemic tradition is provided by attachment theory. Attachment theory does not pathologize dependency in our close relationships. Bowlby (1988) understood that we learn how to know our own minds clearly and straightforwardly with the help and support of a trusted other, and research suggests it does only need to be one other person (Miculincer & Goodman, 2006)—and often this person is the therapist. If we have learned not to trust others because of past hurts and neglect, the therapist acts as the bridge into new, albeit tentative, trusting relationships. Thus, autonomy and dependency are seen as different sides of the same attachment relationship. It is recognized that adults as well as children need emotional security to thrive and that our self-protective attachment strategies will impact and be impacted by our relationships. We suggest that the field of systemic relational therapy with its emphasis on communication, reflexivity, cultural context, narrative, problem solving, and collaboration is deepened in an integration with attachment theory as a theory of love. This then helps to contextualize, conceptualize, and scaffold (in the Vygotskyan sense) the development of connection and emotional bonding in the systemic therapeutic process.

Emotions are relational experiences. They are the fabric of our social lives, reflecting our ability to appraise the state of the other, their needs, and so on. Our affect system helps us navigate love and hate, cooperation and conflict, healing and repair in our relationships, living and dying together. Bowlby understood that our emotions are organized, given meaning, and shaped in the context of our interpersonal relationships, and especially our close relationships. Stern (1985) suggested that our emotions—joy, surprise, excitement, and anger, fear, sadness, envy, and disgust—can only make sense in a relational context.

Attachment theory is a developmental theory of the social regulation of emotion in family systems, with an emphasis on co-regulation. Our attachment systems—that is, our learned self-protective strategies—are activated under conditions of threat and loss, real, imagined, and feared. If the danger is external, the child learns to seek proximity and safety, but sometimes the threat and the danger come from within the family. Children and adults adapt in conditions of relational danger; for example, where a child's understandable negative feelings can threaten the relationship with the caregiver, the process of adaptation and accommodation can lead to the minimizing of the significance of feelings as a good guide to action. Ainsworth, in her research, added the concept of embodied 'felt security', where the child who is motivated to avoid fear and threat and to seek an internal sense of comfort and warmth, experiences the good feelings called love. Arietta Slade, in personal communication with R. Bowlby (1988), notes that John Bowlby latterly called attachment theory a theory of love (in Holmes & Slade, 2017).

The therapeutic relationship can be described and defined as a multi-layered attachment process, encompassing our dispositional representations of love as intention, thought, feeling and sensation, and action. In the safety of the therapeutic relationship, we can learn to both integrate and re-integrate disconnected aspects of difficult experiences, where a lack of integration is impeding our wish for an intimate connection with others and/or a significant other. The goal of therapy is self and relational reflexivity where we assist people to know their own minds, to stand in the emotional shoes of the other, and to listen non-defensively when difficult moments, feelings, and experiences are broached. Non-defensive listening, with the help and support of the therapist, is a complex set of skills that paves the way for apology, healing, and repair. Many of the individuals, couples, and family groups we engage therapeutically suffer from the distress of unresolved hurt and loss in their close relationships, past and present. Resolution does not necessarily make people feel better, as such, but helps to develop a sense of agency and relational responsiveness (response-able) that enables arousal co-regulation, openness to novelty, and more effective decision making (Miculincer & Goodman, 2006).

Some family members have not experienced sensitive and attuned relational boundaries in their childhoods, perhaps because of sexual or other forms of childhood abuse or neglect. They have developed self-protective and defensive strategies to survive into adulthood. In the relationship with the therapist, family members can learn that they are entitled to safety in their close relationships and that they too can boundary what is appropriate and acceptable for them. In the safety of the therapy, family members can experiment and go beyond what has been possible at home.

However, when the person who hurt and abused you was also the one who cared for you, we learn that comfort and care are paired with danger. This presents one of the greatest challenges for therapy—for the therapist, the family members, and all their relationships. The effects of relational danger can be deadening. We work to help people restore and ground themselves, both personally and inter-personally, without overwhelming them. Slow pacing and lengthier therapeutic times are often needed (Vetere & Sheehan, 2017).

The Meeting of Minds

Guntrip (1953), one of the earliest shapers of the family-systemic framework, was one of the first psychotherapists to use the word 'agape' to describe the kind of parental love that therapists offer and create with their clients, the felt safety for family members to practise relating in more satisfying ways, to assist with 'making the unknown known' (Wallin, 2010). Ringrose (2014) writes that it is in the consistency of the therapist's warmth, love, and care that clients can form strong enough bonds that challenge unhelpful assumptions about self, others, and relationships. The special challenge for systemic therapists is to create balanced loving relationships with more than one person in the room, in ways that leave no one person feeling unseen and unheard.

Daniel Stern (2004) describes 'now moments'—when hearts and minds are working together—no words may need to be spoken—when therapist and client/s gaze at each other in a felt and mutual understanding and feelings of warmth and love flow between them. Stern suggests that in these 'now moments', we experience our greatest potential for learning and growth. We suggest that this also includes the development of the therapist. Therapist disclosure in therapy is not self-exposure. The self-reflexive practitioner grasps the difference between their mind and the minds of their clients and is capable of showing sadness at the pain of the other, and of feeling sad because they cannot always take that pain away. In the moments of self-disclosure, we are sharing something real about ourselves in order to help our clients accept something real, a feeling or an event, in their own lives. This is critical for the client and is an exchange that goes beyond empathy. It is a form of warranting/respecting what they have experienced and endured. This is in service of our client/s and our therapeutic work together; it is not for the therapist. Hearts and minds in our work, no separation of the personal and professional, we do not leave ourselves or our values at the therapy room door. But we do respect the needs of our clients, and our task is to assist. The benefits to us include a deep sense of satisfaction, our ongoing development and learning, and the evolution of our thinking and values, all of which impacts the variety of different roles we occupy in our personal and professional lives.

Many researchers have shown a recursive link between our self-protective strategies in the face of relational danger and our linguistic/narrative ability to communicate a real/true story of ourselves and our experiences rather than a minimized, dismissed, or distorted account (Crittenden & Landini, 2011). This has nothing to do with the ability to talk about ourselves, as such, but is more concerned with how we can story and communicate our experiences of loss, rejection, grief, and pain. It is with love that we help people recognize the reality of their own experiences, their relational needs, to be thoughtful of the feelings and thoughts of others, and to develop a sense of agency that allows them/us to take responsibility for their/our intentions and action. In therapy, we help people resolve the seemingly unresolvable dilemmas and conflicts from their earlier life, with care, concern, and comfort at the leading edge of a healing relationship. But, sadly, when people cannot be curious about their own minds and have learned never to trust others, despite all our best intentions, we all must live with that sense of disappointment that arises when even the best efforts of therapists and clients over the long term do not seem to bear fruit.

Supervision and Therapist Self-Care

The therapist always needs to pay attention to their self-care, and an important part of this happens through the supervision process and the relationship with the supervisor. Earlier in this chapter, we drew attention to some of the negative consequences that arise for therapeutic practice when love is forgotten or sidelined in favour of other variables. Supervision remains one of the chief antidotes to this forgetfulness by helping supervisees to be as present as possible to their clients in their pain, despair, and helplessness. Supervisors can do this by showing up as fully as possible in their supervisory relationships and assisting their supervisees to bear their own pain, despair, and helplessness.

We might say there is so much distress and oppression in the world that if we try to make everything better we risk becoming overwhelmed and thus could burn out (Vetere & Stratton, 2016). Therapeutic and supervisory loving is not without risk. We were never promised a rose garden. But, if we try to protect ourselves from significant pain, perhaps because of own resonance, we will probably not be as fully present and listening as we might be. In acts of self-love, we try to attend to our own feelings of connection and disconnection and how they might shift, subtly, perhaps daily, contextually, and relationally. It is an important question as to how we balance ourselves and remain open, present, and focused, with sufficient energy to engage with others and maintain deepening connections. One aspect of the supervisory role is to help us with this balance—to observe, to challenge, to support, and sometimes to explore the fear of that part of ourselves that family members might represent. It is our belief that family members respond when they know their therapist can bear to hear.

Conclusion

This chapter has sought to reposition the place of love within the therapeutic relationship and to bring it right to the centre, the place where we believe it belongs. We have suggested that love within the therapeutic relationship belongs to that tradition of thinking about love associated with the concept of agape. Against the background of the concept's appearance within psychoanalysis and related therapeutic modalities, we have pursued a distinctively systemic view of agape by considering several reflections of, or windows upon, agape already present within the systemic tradition. We have found these reflections in certain dialogical practices, in systemic therapy's commitment to the exploration of the operation of power and difference, in the perspective on therapy as an attachment process, and in those perspectives that emphasize the meeting of hearts and minds in the present moment. And, finally, we have drawn attention to the important role supervision can and does play in keeping love, in all its complexities, challenges, and healing capacities, alive and growing in the lives of clients, therapists, and supervisors.

References

Andersen, T. (1992). Reflections on reflecting with families. In S. McNamee & K. Gergen (Eds.), *Therapy as a social construction*. Sage.

Bowlby, J. (1988). *A secure base*. Basic Books.

Buber, M. (1988) *The knowledge of man: Selected essays* (M.S. Friedman & R.G. Smith, Trans.). Humanities Press.

Burnham, J. (2005). Relational reflexivity: A tool for socially constructing therapeutic relationships. In C. Flaskas, B. Mason, & P. Perlesz (Eds.), *The space between: Experience, context, process in the therapeutic relationship*. Routledge.

Castonguay, L., Constantino, M., & Holtforth, M. (2006). The working alliance: Where are we and where should we go? *Psychotherapy: Theory, Research, Practice and Training, 43*, 271–279.

Crittenden, P., & Landini, A. (2011). *Assessing adult attachment: A dynamic maturational approach to discourse analysis*. Norton.

Ferenczi, S. (1932). Confusion of tongues between adults and the child: The language of tenderness and of passion. In J. M. Masson (Ed.), *The assault on truth: Freud's suppression of the seduction theory, Appendix C* (pp. 291–303). Ballantine.

Gergen, K. (1996). Technology and the self: From the essential to the sublime. In T. Grodin & T. Lindlof (Eds.), *Constructing the self in a mediated world*. Sage.

Gibran, K. (1923). *The prophet.* Knopf.

Guntrip, H. (1953). The therapeutic factor in psychotherapy. *British Journal of Medical Psychology, 26,* 115–132.

Holmes, J., & Slade, A. (2017). *Attachment in therapeutic practice.* Sage.

Jordan, J., Kaplan, A. G., Miller, J. B., Stiver, I. P., & Surrey, J. L. (1991). *Women's growth in connection.* Guilford.

Lago, C., & Charura, D. (Eds.). (2016). *The person-centred counselling and psychotherapy handbook: Origins, developments and clinical applications.* McGraw Hill.

Lambert, K. (1973). Agape as a therapeutic factor in analysis. *Journal of Analytic Psychology, 18*(1), 25–46.

Loewald, H. W. (1980). Psychoanalytic theory and psychoanalytic process. In H. W. Loewald (Ed.), *Papers on psychoanalysis* (pp. 227–301). Yale University Press.

Lothane, Z. (1996). In defense of Sabina Spielrein. *International Forum of Psychoanalysis, 5,* 203–217.

Lothane, Z. (1998). The feud between Freud and Ferenczi over love. *The American Journal of Psychanalysis, 58*(1), 21–39.

Maturana, H. R., & Varela, F. J. (1987). *The tree of knowledge: The human biological roots of understanding.* New Science Library.

Miculincer, M., & Goodman, G. (2006). *Dynamics of romantic love: Attachment, care-giving and sex.* Guilford.

Minuchin, S. (1974). *Families and family therapy.* Harvard Univ. Press.

Munoz-Martinez, A. M., & Follette, W. C. (2019). When love is not enough: The case of therapeutic love as a middle-level term in functional analytic psychotherapy. *Behaviour Analysis: Research and Practice, 19*(1), 103–113.

Ringrose, J. (2014). Psychotherapy for disorganised attachment, dissociation, and dissociative identity disorder. In D. Charura & S. Paul (Eds.), *The therapeutic relationship handbook: Theory and practice.* OU Press.

Rogers, C. R. (1992). The necessary and sufficient conditions of therapeutic personality change. *Journal of Consulting and Clinical Psychology, 60,* 827–832.

Sanday, W., & Headam, A. C. (1908). *A critical and exegetical commentary on the epistle to the Romans.* T. and T. Clark.

Satir, V. (1988). *The new people-making.* Science and Behaviour Books.

Seikkula, J., & Trimble, D. (2005). Healing elements of therapeutic conversation: Dialogue as an embodiment of love. *Family Process, 44*(4), 461–475.

Seikkula, J., Aaltonen, J., Alakare, B., Haarakangas, K., Keranen, J., & Sutela, M. (1995). Treating psychosis by means of open dialogue. In S. Friedman

(Ed.), *The reflective team in action: Collaborative practice in family therapy* (pp. 62–80). Guilford.

Snyder, M. (2000). Mutual love in the therapeutic process. *Journal of Systemic Therapies, 19*(4), 4–19.

Stern, D. (1985). *The interpersonal world of the infant.* Routledge.

Stern, D. (2004). *The present moment in psychotherapy and everyday life.* Norton.

Tsai, M., Callaghan, G. M., & Kohlenberg, R. J. (2013). The use of awareness, courage, therapeutic love and behavioural interpretation in functional analytic psychotherapy. *Psychotherapy, 50*, 366–370.

Vetere, A., & Sheehan, J. (Eds.). (2017). *Long term systemic therapy.* Palgrave Macmillan.

Vetere, A., & Stratton, P. (Eds.). (2016). *Interacting selves: Personal and professional development in counselling and psychotherapy.* Routledge.

Wallin, D. (2010). *Attachment in psychotherapy.* Guilford Press.

3

Trust, Movement and Collaboration: An Exploration of Trust, Its Significance and Its Forms of Expression in Therapy Sessions

Tone Grøver and Inger-Margrete Svendsen

Dear Reader

The starting point for this chapter is the experiences we have had over the course of many years as therapists working with couples, families and individuals. In our conversations, we sometimes experience special moments or situations that are perceived as significant, moving and perhaps formative. These are moments that are accompanied by a certain atmosphere in the room and between us who are there, an atmosphere which we would like to bring to light and explore here.

T. Grøver (✉)
Department of Family Therapy and Systemic Practice, Faculty of Social Studies, VID Specialized University, Oslo, Norway
e-mail: tone.grover@vid.no

I.-M. Svendsen
Management, Organization & Growth, Oslo, Norway
e-mail: ingersv2@online.no

© The Author(s), under exclusive license to Springer Nature Switzerland AG 2023
T. Grover et al. (eds.), *New Horizons in Systemic Practice with Adults*, Palgrave Texts in Counselling and Psychotherapy, https://doi.org/10.1007/978-3-031-30526-9_3

Some of these experiences we recall particularly well because they have become significant to us as therapists, and we have had a sense that they have meant something to those who have been our collaboration partners in the therapy room. When we examined these situations more closely, we were struck by the thought that they all seemed to revolve around trust in some way. We also came to wonder at the many different ways in which trust can be expressed, and at how much it demands of both parties. What we would like to emphasize here is the significance of trust and how we manage it in our role. And we would like to bring up the question of whether the many forms and facets of trust can be seen as the very axis of the interaction's orientation in systemic therapy.

From systemic theory, we know something about what creates trust. But this is mostly at a somewhat general level, such as the meaning of listening, accepting, respecting and fostering equality. However, we wish to be even more specific, looking at micro-situations and the subtleties of little sequences, where much of our experience lies, and ask: What is it that gives rise to trust? What are the forms of expression of trust?

Trust is a complex term, and it is difficult to say anything general and precise about it. Trust carries within itself expectations of another person, about what might happen in a given situation. Trust carries within it an expectation that something good will happen, or that a person or group of people wishes me well. To grant trust is thus to be in a vulnerable position. "The defensibility of trust depends on the trustworthiness of others" (translated from Grimen, 2009, pp. 21–22). Thus, we may say that trust or mistrust is gained through experience with the other party, the group or society.

This Chapter's Invitation to You

As we go on to explore trust in the following pages, we would like to invite you as the reader into the exploration of trust in the context of therapy. We will do this by asking you questions along the way. Perhaps you will see something different than we do?

Nils Christie has expressed the following:

> Among the most important is to upgrade people's own experiences, helping people explore their own experiences, make the experiences valid and thereby make the bearer of the experience more secure. Secure in the knowledge that they, through their lives, have experienced something important, something which allows them to understand adjoining subjects, thereby granting them the right to speak up in many arenas. (translated from Christie, 2009, p. 53)

We take this as an encouragement to trust in experience—ours, yours, and that of those who seek our help as therapists.

When we share our experience with you as a reader, we use the subject *I*, even though we are two people writing together based on different personal experiences. In this way, we wish to experiment with highlighting the systemic idea that in every *I*, there is a *we*. The following little dialogue took place when we made this choice. One said: "But I, for instance, am divorced. You are not, in fact you are in your fortieth year of marriage. In this aspect, you are not in my *I*." The other replied: "I, too, am divorced. I have experienced being divorced from others many times. Don't we, therefore, share the experience of being connected, divorced and separated? Aren't I, too, a part of your marital divorce through the way in which we have related to it together?" This seemed to us both like a systemic and ethical perspective which liberated us from the individual *I* in the writing process, while we no longer need to erase personal experiences or keep them isolated to our individual selves. There arose for us a sense of freedom and community, and of not being separate egos. Furthermore, we call those who seek our help our collaboration partners rather than patients. We collaborate on creating movement. Human beings are born to collaborate, as when the little child—before it is able to talk or walk—says "aah" and points to the place where the child wants us to direct our attention, thus making an invitation to collaboration (Tetzcher, 2012). The form of collaboration will of course be different from moment to moment and our question to ourselves and to you is: What is the significance of trust in all of this?

"Show, Don't Tell" and the Refinement of Knowledge About Oneself

A man in his 30s attends therapy sessions. He describes the discomfort and unease he experiences when his girlfriend sets the table for a romantic dinner. There are napkins, candles and quiet music. His discomfort makes it difficult to sit still, difficult to look her in the eyes the way she is hoping he will. It all ends in disappointment, tears and broken expectations—again and again, and he despairs being able to accommodate her needs. He doesn't want to pretend to enjoy intimate dinners with her as he says this would be unauthentic.

I ask: "Does the discomfort remind you of anything? Is it a discomfort you have experienced before?" "Yes," he replies, "it reminds me of having supper at home growing up, of all things." He tells me about the kitchen of his childhood home. And Mom, who wouldn't sit down with him. She remained standing, arms crossed, and watched him eat. This was the only time of day when he could have Mom to himself, without his little siblings. He was slim and meagre and in the story he's about seven years old. He asked: "May I have another slice of bread, Mom?" He got one. When he had eaten it, he asked: "May I have another slice, Mom?" She cut the bread efficiently, spreading the butter with quick motions. She handed it to him with a firm "Here you go". He was so full, almost sick, but again he asked: "May I have another slice, Mom?" While telling me the story, he abruptly stops here, exclaiming: "Don't say anything!" He understood something, I understood something. Neither of us can know whether we understood the same thing. And if he hadn't asked me to stay quiet, I probably would have said something. The danger is that I might have said something that could bring up a connection between the experience then and the experience now.

What happens when we try to draw connections, try to go above and beyond in our role, by providing insight or associations? What might happen, if we leave it up to our conversation partner to let the impressions from their own words and stories remain without trying to accommodate or make further inquiries? Does this touch on questions of trust?

In conversations where difficult experiences are offered up, an important orientation for therapists can be to assist the one we are talking to, in getting a sense of him- or herself. What this man is describing surrounding the romantic dinner sounds to me like a feeling of losing the sense of self. This unpleasant feeling is what Holmgren (2019) calls "everyday dissociation"—which we can all get a taste of in certain situations. He knew me, and clearly didn't want my follow-up questions. Would they be able to disturb his confidence in his own knowledge about himself? Haven't we all experienced that we can become aware of something of importance to ourselves which we can't express with words? And neither can others?

In fiction writing, there is a rule that says "show, don't tell". Working together in a therapy room can be a matter of forming stories and creating meaning from events. Can we, in our roles, be too eager to co-create stories, put words or explanations to what comes, and thereby undermine "show" for the benefit of "tell"? When the subject is trust, and trust in one's own knowledge about oneself, this seems to me like an important question for therapy. This was highlighted in my conversations with a woman who disappeared from our appointments for a while because she got an offer for free therapy through her employer. After a while, she returned with the following frustration: "There was so much explaining. It was exhausting."

What struck me was that I, when talking to this woman, often resorted to explanations. There is something about her that appears tender to me, in some strange way appealing to my need for explanations. As she said this, I wondered if both I, and perhaps the other therapist, were responding to what we *imagine* is something tender, and such interpretations can easily represent a hierarchy in the conversation. *I* am trying to help *you* with *my* knowledge.

During my own years in therapy, I experienced how explanations, which easily come to represent a hierarchy of knowledge, can create uncertainty in my own knowledge about myself, but also what an exquisite tightrope walk this is. It was at times truly redemptive that my therapist suggested words to describe my experiences. At other times, I wished she would refrain from doing so. And how nice it could be when she did exactly that. I once presented her with a mental image: I'm five years old and hiding in a dark closet. My mother and siblings had gone to the movies without me, I was too little to go with them. As a consolation, I had been given a box of pastilles. In the next room, my father was occupied with the writing of some reports; he was completely lost in his work while drinking a glass of vodka. A glass that would make him a little bit different. I remember putting my little finger into the box, fishing out a black, salty pastille, putting it in my mouth, and sucking and sucking. Until the box was empty. The image is perhaps low in significance on one level, but not to me. To me, a sense of loneliness comes to life, which I am unable to precisely articulate, other than through this image. And the image gave me a sense of warmth for myself. My therapist said nothing. But I was a little worried that she would, as it would disturb my own discovery. How can such a simple little image create so much of a sense of myself?

I believe what my two collaboration partners conveyed to me is of great value. And perhaps I have become more attentive to their message due to my own experience: The importance of holding ourselves back in our roles in order to let our collaboration partner gain trust in their own knowledge of him- or herself while also knowing that help is sometimes redemptive. Can we as therapists appeal to our own musicality in this art form of conversation? When faced with the balance between being someone who can offer up words, find connections and help create good narratives and staying silent, can we allow the metaphor or story told to live as the person's knowledge of him- or herself? What are your experiences? What does the rule "show, don't tell" mean to you in your work?

Moving the Perspective

A woman who comes to me for therapy sessions is working with a childhood where the father's alcohol abuse was the axis around which everything revolved. He drank a lot. Every day. She told me how her father was absent, with intoxication dictating his actions. She told me that she had grown up without contact with her father, and how the father's absence became her loneliness. She was sad, disappointed and angry at her father who had ruined the family, who had created a family that was always quarrelling. We talked about her own loneliness when she, as a little girl, hid under the table when the words between the adults became too hard, too violent, flying through the room like knives. She told me that she never dared initiating romantic relationships as an adult because she was unable to trust anyone. She was lonely and longing at the same time. She wanted a relationship but also pushed all opportunities away. She said she "trusts no one", while she was sharing, and her trust lay between us like a thin veil. My collaboration partner cried and raged, and something lightened from seeing the source of the pain, yet there was something that wouldn't let go.

When I went to see her again, I had been thinking about the prison she had described, about the fact that something wouldn't let go despite her gaining insight into the source of the pain and working with it. This is something I see often. It's as though insight is not always enough. Perhaps this is a pain point in therapy. I wanted to introduce a new perspective. I think therapy can be about making hypotheses, trying out different approaches to see if something creates movement. We boldly go forth and see what happens.

I wanted to try moving the attention from the individual to the surrounding contextual factors and wondered if this could help. What do you think about that? What experiences can you draw on as a therapist when it comes to bringing up contextual circumstances?

After a little while in this conversation, I asked: "Can you see any connections between your father's alcohol abuse and his life circumstances?" After a pause, she said: "Yes, yes, he came from harsh conditions, poverty, his father [my interlocutor's grandfather] had been violent to my grandmother." After a period of silence, she continued: "Maybe there's something here? Has my father been trying to cope with life through the alcohol? I have been laying all the blame on him alone and I can feel that I still wish to do that."

Me: "Yes, I can understand that. After all, he and your mother were responsible for creating good conditions for you and your siblings growing up. I empathize with your sentiment and don't mind us holding on to it."

Her: "Yes, perhaps, but we have worked a lot on processing all the painful experiences. Maybe the time has come to … I don't know … look at him?"

Me: "Yes, maybe. I am sometimes focused on broadening the perspective—but this may not be right for you, or it may be the wrong time for it. I sometimes proceed too quickly—this I know. So, I'm happy to have you stop me."

Her: "But he's a human being, too. He's probably been imprisoned by his own experiences, too. By his class, which was characterized by masculine violence and alcohol to cope with life. They worked and they drank. He was a very proud man."

Me: "A proud man you say, tell me more."

Her: "He was very handsome in his youth, strong, he worked as a construction worker and was dutiful. He was well liked at his workplace and had a booming laugh. I was always so glad to hear that laugh, and I can still hear it in my head."

Me: "How nice to hear—I can almost picture him."

Her: "Hmm. That felt strange, telling you about him. I haven't thought about it like that before. Maybe he drank to endure his rough memories and experiences, the hard life at work, financial problems, failing to give us kids what we needed, his aching body. Maybe this was defeat to him? I myself can barely endure what I've been through, maybe he couldn't endure what he'd been through? Maybe enduring himself as a violent man demanded that he be intoxicated? He must have suffered, that man. I haven't thought about him that way before."

Me: "What happens to you when you think like that and ask so many important questions?"

Her: "It all expands, in a way. It's as though something lets go of me. I see him more clearly as a fighter."

Me: "Yes, the image becomes clearer in some sense, and the conditions of life become clearer. We often forget the importance of social circumstances in our lives."

She replied: "You know, this is the first time I feel, as an adult, that I also like my father. I feel bad for him, and I feel a fondness for him, in spite of all the crap he has made me endure. I'm going to go visit him and give him a hug."

She laughed, gave me a hug and left. She went to visit her father.

I remained in my office. I heard her pace quickly down the corridor and disappear. I looked at my watch, she had left ten minutes before our appointment was over. She left in a flash, it was as though a tornado had come into my office. What happened here? What do you think happened when she met her father? What's important here?

I've thought a lot about this since I haven't seen her again. Was it forgiveness? Or is something entirely different happening here? Was it a hug in kindness because she saw him in a greater context? Or was it the recognition that they're both suffering, an empathy for her father that doesn't necessarily lead to forgiveness, but perhaps to peace? Maybe she sees herself when seeing the other, in this case, her father. Maybe this is freedom sometimes? Does redemption lie in seeing the meaning of class, or is it more of an existential bodily acknowledgement of seeing her father's suffering? I have wondered whether she has an "aha moment" when she sees her father as a victim, as she has seen and felt herself as a victim. And does this recognition create action and power?

This makes me wonder whether we sometimes, even in systemic therapy, under-communicate or disregard class and other social and cultural factors. We may then be at risk of forgetting the context of the lives we are living. What kind of trust is necessary in order that the bringing in of a greater perspective, when faced with a person who views their own life as ruined by another, is not received as disapproval?

Suicide: Caring

I would like to share another moment with you, revolving around a situation where the person sitting in front of me is so tormented by painful thoughts and feelings that they see no other solution than suicide. Very often, there are many experiences and events layer upon layer in people who wish to die, disappear or get a respite from the darkness, the blackness, the unendurable.

What happens to me when I am in this situation? What happens to you?

I get scared and feel like I want to escape from the situation. I've noticed that I feel the need to find a solution and become a therapist who shows the way. I have thought this might give hope, but also see that it has probably been a defence mechanism on my part. I feel a strong sense of unease and fear that the person in front of me will die. I would take it as a defeat even though I know, rationally speaking, that there are many factors that carry more weight than those experiences we create together in the room.

As a therapist, I have searched for approaches that can help me keep us together through the pain—not running away from it but accepting it. Help me gain trust for my partner and myself.

A young man of about 25 years of age has been coming to me for sessions for a long time. He struggles with heavy thoughts, a feeling of being broken, experience with a mother who has alternately criticized and praised without him understanding what he was doing to deserve either. He is frustrated and angry. He feels sick of himself and has tried to self-medicate with drugs. It hasn't worked and he feels powerless. We have worked with his experiences over a long period and at times he has been better; he put the drugs aside, resumed his academic pursuits and got a girlfriend—only to have past experiences catch up with him, being filled by heavy, self-destructive thoughts and emotions. This vicious cycle had taken different shapes throughout our period of working together.

One day, he came and sat down in front of me with a serious look on his face. He looked at me with his clear, blue eyes and said: "It's enough. We have worked together for a long time, you and I, and it's been nice. I've received the help I need. I've felt that life can give me something good. Thank you." I felt my heart beating hard and fast. I felt scared. What is he saying? Where is he going with this? What should I say? Thoughts and feelings race through me. I really want to say, as I usually have in similar situations; "Yes, how important, you have felt that life can give you something good. Tell me about those experiences!" Something is holding me back. Is it the serious expression on his face? Is it the "thank you"?

I say: "Yes, we have worked for a long time, we have gone into many of the experiences in your life, it has provided many experiences for the two of us together in this room."

He says: "Hmm. It has, and it all just repeats itself. It catches up with me time and again. I'm tired. I no longer believe I can have a good life."

Me: "You've lost hope?"

Him: "Yes. I have. I only wish to die now, I think about it all the time. I think it's the right thing for me and for my family. I cause them pain, I'm a piece of shit to them, a source of worry, you see?"

Me: "I think I sense your despair in myself and in the room now."

I look at him. He meets my gaze after a while. The seriousness of the situation trembles between us. I let it tremble, holding him with my gaze. He looks down. Weeps.

Me: "I understand so well that you lose hope. You have worked really hard to escape from your past experiences, your powerlessness. The experience of being caught up with by your past, time after time, creates a need for escaping all the pain. This makes sense, Tom."

Silence. He looks out the window before his eyes meet mine.

I ask: "Have you lost all hope or is there some left?"

He says: "When you ask it's as though there's some hope there, just now. It was good, saying it, good that you don't run away and get scared of me."

Here I could have said: "I *am* scared." Could this have reaffirmed my trust that he matters to me? I pick another option, without saying that one is any more right than the other.

I sit at the edge of my seat, turn my whole body towards his and look at him intensely, seriously, with warmth in my voice and say: "I would very much like to continue working with you, if you would give it one more chance? I like you, and you matter to me. If you want to see me again it will be on one condition, which is that you do NOT take your own life while the two of us are in contact. Can you promise me that?"

He says: "Yes…" (some doubt in his voice).

Pause.

He says: "Yes, I want that. I want that."

I get up and squat down in front of him and reach out my hand. We shake hands and look at each other. We hold hands and affirm a promise.

How do you interpret this sequence? What might happen here?

After we have understood and gained contact with the pain, given meaning to the sense that suicide might feel like a "solution", this approach has given me and the other enough peace to continue working together. I feel scared in such situations, and the way to keep a hold of the contact and the gravity of the situation is to trust in our mutual cooperation. That we have something here which we stand in and affirm with our agreement. I also reach for the existential subject by saying, "I like you. You matter to me." I don't say this as an instrumental approach but as a truly felt condition within me. Like the reciprocal character of agapic love mentioned by Sheehan and Vetere (2023, this volume), I have the experience of being nourished and touched by Tom.

To "matter" is at the heart of life, mattering to oneself, to others, to something beyond oneself. Is the sense of not mattering the very core of the suicidal idea? I dare to believe, and trust, that the sentence "You matter to me" can be translated to and felt as "I (in this case Tom) matter". Could this be a basis for existential meaning beyond this relationship and situation? As Nils Christie asks, in the introductory quote?

An underlying theme in the collaborative effort we call therapy is complementarity. One is the helper and one (or more if it is couples or families) needs help, one is there in a professional capacity and the other is not. Then a relevant question could be: do you really care as a person or is it the role that cares? Or might it be the method that creates a veil of apparent caring? Are we faced with an ethical challenge here? Are we bound to be overinvolved by caring as human beings? Has the term "professional distance" come in as a defence against this? Does it help you in your work? Or does it hinder you? Is being present and caring as a human being a prerequisite for movement?

To me, caring is a way of being vital, creative and alive. It helps me hold on to concentration, presence and meaning when faced with other people. It also reminds me of my own life and life processes. Much of the discussion surrounding the lives of therapists suggests that being too involved is draining and must be limited. Does this discussion affect the trust we are able to build in the therapy room? Where is the creative balance between intimacy and distance?

What Creates Trust When Different Considerations Are in Opposition?

A father comes to therapy sessions with two of his three adult sons. The sons are angry with their father, and they carry a lot of anger in general. They are tired of themselves and their own anger, they despair of it, they find themselves verbally losing control of themselves, and it affects their own wives and children. They have been struggling with this—and their own father is struggling with their anger. He has been convinced that something is wrong with his sons. In our conversations, the sons repeatedly get angry at their father. The father despairs, he says he is scared to open his mouth, it'll be wrong no matter what he says. One of the sons says:

> You have to start caring about yourself, Father. You completely lack self-reflection. It's all run by your bookish head. You have no sense of yourself or us, no wonder you don't understand your own missteps. You can't have had an easy time with Grandma and Grandpa. They were so cold!

> The father: "I think I had a good childhood. Yes, in fact, I had a very nice upbringing. And I was grateful for all the love I received."

Do questions of trust arise in this micro-situation which also concern me and my role? I believe so, and the questions are complex. The son is in one way trying to build trust in his father by showing insight into the father's life. At the same time, there is a criticism baked in with what he is saying, which might awaken the defence mechanisms in the father. In any case, the father takes the son's statement as something he wants to correct. Is there also a criticism, or a piece of advice, within the father's words? Perhaps hinting that he, as opposed to his sons, was grateful for what he got as a child? It *can* be interpreted this way. And this is how I hear it. What are my responsibilities if I am to hold firm the idea that without trust nothing of value will be created in this room? If I let this pass, do I contribute to a weakening of the son's trust in his father? Or of me? Or worse: The son's trust in himself and his own judgement? I know it can be tempting to give up on conversations like this when it seems like there is no hope of getting through to the other. If I don't react, this could be taken as confirmation that it is *right* to give up because I let it pass. In conversations, we often lack the time for pondering such questions because the moments pass, leaving their marks. It is our responsibility to listen for what is important, and sometimes latch onto it. In this particular instance, I stop the father and ask:

"What do you think happens with your son, when you say you were grateful for the love you received?"

The father: "I have no idea, how should I know?"

Me: "Do you suppose he might take this to mean he should be just as grateful as you were?"

Father: "But that's not what I meant, I *was* grateful."

The son erupts. He says this is exactly how it is. It is impossible to get through. It is impossible to speak earnestly with his father, who is only playing games, in the interest of raising his sons in his own image. At the same time, I notice how grateful the son is for my challenging the father, in this little sequence of which they have so many. The father ends up in the "corner of shame", with a double shame because he doesn't understand. The son and I feel an alliance. Is this right or wrong of me? Does it bring trust, or break it down? Isn't it in such little sequences that relationships are built, trust is created, broken down or put to the test? I see it as our task precisely to be attentive to the subtle messages. These are the building blocks of relationships but can be perceived as "too insignificant" for those affected to take action. And we should be wary of what the power we possess in our role might create from micro-moment to micro-moment (Oddli et al. 2021; White 2000, 2007). How can I justify what I do in this little scene?

We can easily be paralyzed in conversations if we become too scared of destroying trust. And if we are paralyzed, or become too passive, we may easily end up allowing verbal infringements to happen with our blessing. I still wonder if I am making a shortcut here when I make the choices I do, and refrain from showing the father trust in his own knowledge, which again—who knows—could create what the son is requesting? The son is precisely requesting the father's contact with himself. Who am I to overlook this? Sometimes I find that if I get too impatient, I might end up working against my own project of creating trust in own experience, in the person I am talking to. Upbringings are rarely just good or bad. They are complex for all of us. Thinking about it in retrospect, making a different choice here could have made it easier for the father to grasp what is most important to him as a father, given his knowledge of his own upbringing. Does the choice I actually make have the potential to dig even deeper trenches between father and son? Of course, it would all depend on the character of the further conversation. But it is worth asking why I didn't take the father's statement about his good childhood seriously. Instead, I continued as follows:

> Neither of us should throw the first stone. You and I are in the same boat. I know well how it feels, looking at my own shortcomings, and what they have created for my children. But I wonder if I can also feel myself becoming emotionally crippled if I try to lay blame or responsibility on them? Yes, for my own part, I can feel that. I don't know what you think about that?

This is a wise father. I have no business judging him as either wise or otherwise, of course, but to me he seems wise. He says:

> "I see what you mean. I feel it. I don't understand why I have to defend myself all the time, I'm so tired of it."
>
> Me: "Welcome to the club. At least we are two in it, that's nice to know for me as well."

The choice I make here, partly as a reflex, partly because I am holding on to the systemic idea that we *are* a we, and that there's always a resonance and recognition in what another says, makes me hold on to what I see as a new and creative alliance with the father. In retrospect, I see what opportunities to help him become aware of his own knowledge I thereby let pass. What if I had stopped at his being tired of defending himself? If he is tired of it, it is presumably because there is something else he would rather be doing. What would that be?

In the systemic view, we are cognizant of the fact that we are ourselves a part of the system of those who seek our help. We can't stand outside of it. And perhaps this is part of what drives me to hold on to the resonance I get with the father's experience. But I wonder if this could get in the way of the knowledge the father has about himself and what he cares about.

I don't mind leaving these questions unanswered. But shouldn't we be very attentive to such questions, if we are concerned with trust's many forms of expression? What kind of trust would you wish for in this situation? How would you have liked to be met?

Final Remarks

What we have tried to do in this chapter is to emphasize the significance of trust, and how we manage it, when working with our collaboration partners. The focus of the chapter has been to bring to light the nuances of what trust demands of both parties in the collaboration we are engaged in, which we call therapy. We have attempted to show a few moments of experience to highlight the potential inherent in the subtle little sequences of interaction. Perhaps our lives are shaped precisely—and sometimes radically—in such micro-moments. Through our exploration, we have illuminated our own experiences as well as those of others, and we hope in this way to upgrade the significance of and trust in experiences in our lives.

We could have chosen countless other experiences, and thus shown entirely different sides to the diversity of trust. So, in this way, this chapter can be read as an invitation to trust in your own experiences—and your relationship with trust—as a human being and therapist. Therefore, this is only a first pass, and the continuation could be composed by you and your collaboration partners.

Best regards,

Tone and Inger-Margrete

PS: If you would like, feel free to send us a reply with some thoughts and reflections.

tone.grover@tonegrover.no and ingersv2@online.no

References

Christie, N. (2009). *Små ord for store spørsmål [Small words for big questions]*. Universitetsforlaget.

Grimen, H. (2009). *Hva er tillit [what is trust]*. Universitetsforlaget.

Holmgren, Anette (2019) Komplekse traumers psykologi [The psychology of complex trauma]. DISPUKs forlag.

Sheehan, J., & Vetere, A. (2023). Introduces us to a Systemic View of Agape in therapy. In *New horizon in systemic practice with adults*. Palgrave.

Oddli, H., McLeod, J., Nissen-Lie, H. A., Rønnestad, M. H., & Halvorsen, M. (2021). Future orientation in successful therapies: Expanding the concept of goal in the working alliance. *Journal of Clinical Psychology, 77*(6), 1307–1329. https://doi.org/10.1002/jcip.23108

Tetzcher, v. S. (2012). *Utviklingspsykologi. [Developmental psychology]*. Gyldendal.

White, M. (2000). *Reflections on narrative practice*. Dulwich Centre Publications.

White, M. (2007). *Maps of narrative practice*. WW Norton Co.

4

Questioning Forgiveness

Anne Øfsti and Bård Bertelsen

Under the seams runs the pain
(Anne Carson, *Autobiography of Red*, p. 98)

Prelude (Anne)

As a child, I had a black-and-white photograph on the wall beside my night lamp. It depicted Jesus carrying a lamb over his shoulders. Jesus looked like a movie star, and I remember looking at the picture, praying *please look after mom, dad, my siblings, and me, and please forgive me for not being kind enough.* Many years later, I went through an existential crisis. I could no longer believe in a meta-narrative addressing God as eternally good and fair and Jesus as a saviour who conquered darkness and evil by forgiving all the sins of humankind. What about death, sickness, injustice, unbearable pain, rape, or the rape of children? I could not keep

---

A. Øfsti (✉)
VID Specialized University, Oslo, Norway
e-mail: anne.ofsti@vid.no

B. Bertelsen
University of Agder, Kristiansand, Norway

© The Author(s), under exclusive license to Springer Nature Switzerland AG 2023   **47**
T. Grover et al. (eds.), *New Horizons in Systemic Practice with Adults*, Palgrave Texts in Counselling and Psychotherapy, https://doi.org/10.1007/978-3-031-30526-9_4

believing in an almighty God; this was a loss, and I felt like I had missed the most valuable moral compass in my young life. Still, I kept believing in the importance of forgiveness. I thought of it in terms of *telos*, in the way Aristotle uses that concept to refer to the final purpose of something: the purpose of being human is to forgive, as the purpose of an eye is to see.

Introduction

We, the authors, are clinicians and supervisors, as well as academics. In our years of practising family therapy—Anne first in the Norwegian far north and then, for most of her working years, in Oslo, and Bård in the Agder region in the Norwegian far south—the issue of forgiveness has repeatedly presented itself as a persistent knot. In this chapter, we aim to share some of our experience—one could perhaps even call it expertise (as in "having learnt something from experience"), as it relates to issues of forgiveness.

In relational therapies, at least in a Western, Judeo-Christian tradition, forgiveness is an omnipresent problem. When questions of interpersonal transgression are raised ("You raped me"; "I cheated on you"; "I don't feel loved by you anymore"), they point to a rupture in the social fabric: this used to run smooth, now, it is crinkled. Can it be restored? Should it?

Acknowledging the personal nature of forgiveness, in what follows, we apply autoethnographic means to explore forgiveness as a question that is both cultural, professional-pragmatic, and, at the same time, entirely visceral and subjective. Hence, we presuppose that forgiveness is not first and foremost a general phenomenon but a claim that becomes real, or comes into question, when conceded by a self (an *autos*).

In developing the text and its argument, we have worked in bursts of writing (followed by stretches of non-writing). To preserve some of this textual anatomy, the text is divided into numbered paragraphs. While working with it, our writing punctuated on scenes where forgiveness had emerged as a normative question in our personal histories. To retain the subjective nature of the accounts of these experiences, parts of the text have been written in the voice of the first-person singular. In these parts, the writing subject is indicated in parenthesis.

Alternating between narratives of personal encounters where forgiveness has laid bounds on our experience, insights from other thinkers, and arguments of a more general character, our goal is not to theorise forgiveness in therapeutic terms but rather to dwell with, and illuminate, the fundamental questionability or, perhaps one should rather say the *question-ness*, that lies at the heart of forgiveness: *Can you forgive? Can I?* The following paragraphs are intended to be one possible itinerary for such an undertaking. We suggest that you read them in the order presented, although opting for a different sequence might prove just as rewarding.

II

The word "forgiveness" comes from Old English *forgiefan*, meaning to "give, grant, allow; remit (a debt)", or to "pardon (an offence)", but also to "give up" and "give in marriage". Philosophical accounts of forgiveness often assume that it consists of three components: (1) an overcoming of hostile emotions towards the wrongdoer; (2) a change of heart vis-à-vis the wrongdoer, involving not only the cessation of hostile emotions but also the achievement of a more positive attitude towards her; and (3) a preparedness to restore the relationship and advance towards reconciliation (Verbin, 2010, p. 3).

The normative surge to forgive is strong in Western cultures. Some even claim forgiveness to be a primate instinct (de Waal & van Roosmalen, 1979). By forgiving and repairing relationships, so the theory goes, our ancestors were better positioned to reap the advantages of cooperation between group members, increasing their chances of survival.

According to the philosopher Hannah Arendt, "without being forgiven, released from the consequences of what we have done, our capacity to act would, as it were, be confined to one single deed from which we could never recover; we would remain the victims of its consequences forever" (Arendt, 2018, p. 237). As fallible human beings, we would not be able to get along with each other—as dyads, not to mention as societies—without the capacity, and inclination, to forgive.

But what does the act of forgiving contain? Is forgiveness something one can ask for? If I do something to you that is, as it were, *un*-forgivable—what is it that you do if you decide to forgive it all the same? And if I do not seek forgiveness for my wrongdoings, who—what—am I, then?

III (Bård)

Forgiveness as precept—The tiger and the hedgehog

Years ago, I had a peculiar encounter with animal forgiveness. Or, perhaps what I encountered was not animal at all. Maybe it was simply a projection of normative expectations inscribed in me—a silly fantasy. It is difficult to know. When I was studying psychology at university, I went to a workshop with a shaman proclaiming to be able to take participants on a journey to the Sámi Netherworld to meet their power animals.[1] According to Sámi tradition, life is simultaneously lived in several distinct but interlinked dimensions. What happens in one dimension is not analogously accessible to experience in other dimensions, yet it affects what happens there. In the Netherworld, the power animals of each person live. If something happens to a person's power animal, it can manifest as illness or malaise in the human sphere. Travelling between worlds to observe, and sometimes intervene in what is going on there, is a shaman's gift and obligation.

In the workshop, the shaman placed us participants on our backs on the floor and started to walk among our scattered bodies as he hummed and beat a drum with a frail stick. He instructed us to close our eyes, imagine being in a desolate landscape, and look for a hole in the ground. If we found the hole, we were to jump into it and let ourselves fall through the tunnel into which it led. On the other side of it would be the

---

[1] The concept "power animal" was introduced by Michael Harner in the book *The Way of the Shaman* (Harner, 1980, pp. 57–72). It draws inspiration from animistic practices in cultures from all over the world. In shamanism, power animals are often connected to inner personal growth. They can be contacted with the help of drumming (Boekhoven, 2013, p. 245). See also Äikäs and Fonneland (2021). My story is not meant to represent, nor as an ironisation over, Sámi tradition. I simply tell it in as precise and truthful way as I can, based on memory.

Netherworld. Once there, we were to call out to announce our arrival and summon our power animal.

Listening to the shaman dancing, beating on his drum, and humming faintly, I drifted off into a trance. And, sure enough, while imagining walking through, or hovering over, a tundra-like scenery, I found the hole, jumped in, and soon hit the ground in a strange, bluish, forest-like place on the other side of the tunnel. I yelled out (not truly aloud, I hoped afterwards), "Who will be my power animal?!" and waited. And there, on the edge of a small clearing in the woods, two creatures came walking towards me: a tiger and a hedgehog.

I could tell that the two were not exactly kindred spirits, even from afar. While the hedgehog was strolling peacefully, the tiger seemed noticeably uncomfortable. Once they reached where I was standing, the hedgehog looked straight at me and introduced them as my power animals. From now on, they would remain my faithful companions in this parallel sphere of Sámi reality. He spoke in a soft, relaxed voice, with the faintest of smiles at the edge of his little mouth. Then, the tiger started to speak in an insecure, quivering baritone. He confessed that, literally moments ago, he had eaten every single member of this hedgehog's family. When I called out for them, he was wiping his whiskers from the meal. He assured us—and more the hedgehog than me—that not even in his craziest dreams could he have imagined that the two of them would be teamed up—for *life*, no less. He apologised for creating such an unfortunate beginning to our—from now on eternal—relationship. Glancing sideways at the hedgehog, he retracted his gaze nervously as his tiny partner calmly turned towards him and spoke: "Never mind. You're a tiger. That's the kind of thing tigers do." Then, they turned around and walked away, side by side.

IV

To forgive is not the same as forgetting, psychological denial, or dissociation of a memory. Forgiveness can be an act towards reparation of a relationship, but it does not alter the fact that damage has occurred. In Christian tradition, the ability to forgive is more of a virtue on the victim's part than the end goal of atonement for a perpetrator. Forgiveness frees the one forgiving from being bound by past inflictions.

The philosopher Jacques Derrida (2001) argues that forgiveness, in its Christian form, is not only a salient virtue but also part of a set of values that determine the language of law and politics in our present, globalised community (p. 32).[2] In a world where we constantly step on each other's toes, forgiveness is, in a sense, needed for us to "get on with business". In our interpersonal relationships, just as in the realm of international politics. Forgiveness, when used as a procedure to get to some form of a final end, that is, to a state that we already know and desire, is never "pure", Derrida observes. When forgiveness is taken as a reparative means towards re-establishing normality, forgiving demands a degree of negotiation, or transaction, that inevitably involves a degree of force. Hence, it is impure.

V (Anne)

A mother I knew

I was ten or eleven when a mother told me her stories from her childhood, squeezing a napkin in her hand. I still remember how scared I was, just looking at her. We were always alone. In fact, she would tell me her stories when we were alone. Perhaps she felt a need to, as an explanation for her erratic temper. Or maybe she just had an urgent need to share her pain with me. I remember her telling me *you are listening so well, and I need you to know*. She told me that her parents hated each other. It was an open war between them, from which they never reconciled. As their child, neither did they ever attempt reconciliation vis-à-vis her. To them, there seemed to be nothing to reconcile.

Her mother had been a piano teacher and a conservative Christian. She was surrounded by this dark, ominous atmosphere; every joy in life was a sin, and Doomsday was nearby. In this habitat of scariness and fear, this girl—who was now a mother herself—grew up. Her father was a

---

[2] Derrida uses the term *globalatinisation* to underscore the Roman Christian roots, and contents, of the values disseminated through what is called "globalisation", thus highlighting the Eurocentric, interested nature of globalisation itself.

Don Juan archetype: a doctor, drinking whisky, smoking indoors, enjoying the outdoors, hunting, and fishing—both in a literal and metaphoric sense. Never once did I hear this woman share one pleasant, peaceful memory from her childhood. I never saw a photograph where her family was together. In her stories, they only existed as the persons who destroyed her life and made her vulnerable and often indefinitely ill for long periods. Never healed, she is now in her eighties, suffering from slight dementia. She has told me that she still cries daily over her painful childhood and the absence of comforting memories of care and love. Instead, she became a consumer of self-help literature, hoarding shelves upon shelves of titles promising her a better life. She also went to see a therapist. Once, she said that the only thing she wished for her children was Jesus Christ and psychotherapy.

In my early adult years, I decided to become a family therapist. To me, forgiveness was the pivotal gift of relational life. I still remember how taken I was every time I heard someone say *I forgive you* in the course of a therapy session. Looking back on the ageing woman's story, I wonder how it would have been for her if her parents had come back to ask for her forgiveness. I realise that it could never happen. Since her parents most likely did not see themselves as doing something wrong against their children or being mean or cruel. Harassment within families was not an ethical or moral question in those times. Reconciliation requires, at the very least, some form of awareness that another person has been hurt. Still, I cannot help wondering what would have happened if her parents might have come back from the dead to say, *Please forgive us, we didn't know back then, but now we feel your pain in our hearts, and we can't find peace before you forgive us.* Was it the longing for such a miracle that kept her in therapy? Or made her spend what must have been years of solitary soul searching and fortunes on self-help literature?

In therapy, clients often share heart-breaking dilemmas, making the therapeutic process into a quest that is, ultimately, about existential survival. Some of these quests remain with me after the end of the therapeutic relationship. A while ago, I met with a couple in their mid-fifties. *N* told me that her partner was distant, estranged, and hostile. *M* denied being like that, instead accusing *N* of being jealous, irrational, and neurotic. *N* had developed bodily and mental symptoms, ranging from heart disease and severe infections to panic attacks. *M* finally admitted that he had been involved in a sexual relationship with another woman but assured her that this had ended. He said, "I love you—please forgive me." The reparation should start, but how?

M: We must look forward and move ahead.
N: How?

Some of the most beautiful, nourishing moments in therapy occur when couples are healed from the wounds of past violations, when lack of confidence transforms to trust, comfort, and new beginnings. Often, these processes are made possible by the combination of the passing of time, the careful and precise use of language, addressing guilt and responsibility, and the enactment of hope and humility.

Yet, in my dialogues with this couple, *N* communicated an experience of being too traumatised, bitter, and full of revenge:

M: You must forgive me.
N: I can't.
M: Everyone can forgive, but you don't want to?
N: I know I should, but my body just hurts even more; it is like the word itself is a poisoned knife.

I remember a deep fascination for the fairy tales I was told as a child, especially the use of magic formularies. By saying *Hokus Pokus* or *Abracadabra*, the mountain cracked, the monster vanished, or the empty table was miraculously set. What looked like a dire situation could be transformed into thrilling possibilities using a few seemingly simple words. *Abracadabra—I forgive you.* Looking back at this couple, *M* and *N*, why wouldn't the formula work? *N* said,

"I love him, and I want to do whatever it takes to reconcile, go on, and heal my inner self, but I can't. And I know deep inside that if I could, he and I would have a fair chance of staying together." As a therapist, I kept wondering why she could not just let her resentment go. Not even when she believed that *M*'s adultery belonged to the past and that forgiveness was all that stood between her and the future life that she desired? Are there any keys to understanding the paradox? She said, "Maybe I have too many injuries from childhood." And then she said, "I am losing myself, my sense of self, dignity, and inner strength. I can't take the risk of reconciling. It is not safe."

VI (Bård)

Doing the un-forgivable and discursive rebellion

Therapy, as a general phenomenon, is strongly connected to adverse life events, that is, to things happening in life that are experienced as problematic beyond what is bearable in some way. Since such events often involve other people, forgiveness frequently presents itself as a theme to be dealt with in therapies—bullying, parental involvement (or lack thereof) in an unhappy childhood, infidelity, acts of violence, abuse.

In my practice as a clinical psychologist, I have encountered the issue of forgiveness in numerous contexts. Where it has been most pressing, I believe, was in family-based therapeutic work with young people who had abused other young people sexually. In this work, the fact of a moral transgression (as opposed to presumed symptoms of a disorder or unresolved intra- or interpersonal issues) was always the starting point for therapeutic work. In one conversation with a teenage boy in this context, the issue of forgiveness presented itself thus:

Bård: Those things that you did to that other kid. How do you think they affected him?
Boy: I … I think they broke him.
Bård: Broke him … What do you think about that?
Boy: It's … Just horrible.
Bård: If you were to meet him sometime, and talk to him—is there anything you would like to say to him, do you think?
Boy: I don't know. Probably … Just … to say that none of it was his fault. It was all on me. What happened was my responsibility. It was I who wanted it, not he.

As a therapist, what I most vividly remember from this conversation is the urge I had to ask him if he wanted the other boy—whom he had forced to engage in sexual activities with him on numerous occasions—to forgive him.

> When I finally brought it up, I was surprised by his answer: "No," he said, "I cannot ask that of him. He must be free to do what he needs to do with this. I simply want him to know I am the one to blame."

I have wondered if this boy's stance towards forgiveness shows a different approach to the question of forgiveness than the "impure" urge to re-establish normalcy. According to Derrida (2001), "pure" forgiveness (as an idealised phenomenon) is not, and "*should not be*, normal, normative, normalising. It *should* remain exceptional and extraordinary, in the face of the impossible: as if it interrupted the course of historical temporality" (p. 32, italics in original). Perhaps this boy intuited that forgiveness, in his situation, would be an exception from reality that it was not for him to hope for.

VII

From a relational and psychological viewpoint, forgiveness is a duty and a healthy way to grow as a human. It is so taken for granted that it is nearly impossible to perceive how it could be otherwise. But still, we have a sense of dissent to a doctrine, telling what to do, universally and without context. Why has the imperative about forgiveness been so strong that it feels like a natural law?

A Norwegian philosopher, Arne Johan Vetlesen, asks: *Can it be morally wrong to forgive?* First and foremost, it is a generous thought; we are not alone in struggling with these questions. Vetlesen takes it further, transforming it into a moral question. It is like swearing in the church since the philosophical and religious canons emphasise forgiveness as a duty and virtue. When someone has injured another, it creates an asymmetry. If the victim refuses to forgive, this imbalance will be upheld in the relationship. So, for a future relationship, it is good to balance. Vetlesen discusses, with Kant's Theory of Radical Evil, whether there are actions we neither could punish nor forgive. Vetlesen argues that such actions exist and that the willingness—eagerness to forgive—might evoke future evil actions. A collective emphasis on the virtue of forgiveness could inspire future perpetrators to do evil deeds. Focusing on the actor, which has a "right" to be forgiven, highlights the *person* and takes attention away from the violence. The offender offers prominence—over the evil action. It is essential to take this perspective regarding terror, war, and homicide. But what about less deadly activities? Betrayals, violation, ignorance, domestic violence, and sin of omission?

VIII (Anne)

One afternoon while writing, my laptop suddenly shut down, and I lost a paragraph where I explored my personal processes of reconciliation. I wonder—was there a meaning behind—can technology behave with purpose? Of course not, but still, it allowed me to rethink what would be essential to share. I realised that forgiveness, in my life, has been a speech act of politeness. *Can you forgive me?* equals *I apologise for my bad behaviour and the harm it unintentionally has caused.* But still, I reflect on one experience where I have not held the desire to forgive. And it is a paradox to me. I know others think of me as immature, stubborn, and harsh, since the person that did me harm had only good intentions. It would certainly have made things easier if I were able to forgive. I can recognise the sense of freedom that comes with the thought of letting it go. There is nothing left of trouble in the relationship in question. But in this case, to me, the idea of forgiving is associated with a sense of losing something more valuable than what reconciliation can offer. One explanation is that the harm exposed is so subtle and impossible to name. Hence, I uphold the asymmetry since I do not want a future relationship with this person. I conserve the necessary unrest in my body by not giving in to the urge to forgive. Not-forgiving works as a reminder that hurtful actions harm, even if the offender does not realise that what they are doing is wrong.

Not forgiving keeps me on guard. Hopefully, it sharpens my ability to help clients address unhealthy relationships, almost invisible to those unfamiliar with their kind as such relationships often are. As someone who has felt, and is still feeling, the toil of not forgiving, I hope to be able to deliberately dialogue about the complexity of forgiveness. In the situation of *N* and *M*, they both wanted to heal their relationship and nourish it in the future. Perhaps forgiveness could make the pain melt away in the long run. But for *N*, such an investment seemed to come at enormous costs. What should she do? Who knows?

IX

In *The Cultural Politics of Emotion*, Sara Ahmed (2014) writes that "peace and harmony cannot be linked without the transformation of proximity into a duty that requires others to mimic the very forms of community, which produce violence against others" (p. 199). When proximity and the ability to "get along" are prioritised unquestioningly, the right to refuse to go on or decline the invitation to enter or re-establish relationships is made suspicious.

Forgiving proclaims that, despite what has happened, life can be equally liveable as it used to be. Thus, the (un-)forgivable act is, in a sense, a rupture, a revolt against the order of things, an action that *cannot* be normalised within the existing order. In a sense, forgiveness is the opposite, or, perhaps more precisely, the one-sided dissolution, of conflict.

When we imagine the (un-)forgivable, our imagining works within a discursive horizon—we picture the act to be forgiven as something that we *already* condone. But sometimes, un-forgivables may work the other way, too; on 1 December 1955, in Montgomery, Alabama, Rosa Parks refused to give up her seat in the "coloured" section of a bus, despite being ordered to do so by the driver.[3] For refusing to obey the driver's authority, she was arrested. She was not "forgiven" for her act but punished. Her arrest led to what became known as the Montgomery Bus

---

[3] For details, see https://www.washingtonpost.com/posteverything/wp/2015/12/01/how-history-got-the-rosa-parks-story-wrong/ (accessed 25. June 2022). The inspiration to use the Rosa Parks example comes from reading Gert Biesta's (2020) article "Can the prevailing description of educational reality be considered complete? On the Parks-Eichmann paradox, spooky action at a distance and a missing dimension in the theory of education".

Boycott, lasting for a whole year until a federal ruling was finally implemented, declaring that the Alabama and Montgomery laws about passenger segregation on buses were unconstitutional.

In a sense, this legal reform meant that Rosa Parks was forgiven for what, at the time, had been a violation. But it occurred, notably, not through a process of normalisation but by altering legal reality so that her act (and all other acts like it) was made normal. Precisely because it was un-forgivable within the bounds of the existing order, it provoked the reconfiguration of the order of things itself.

CODA

According to Vetlesen (2007), our most basic and strongest moral experiences stem from offence. Hence, he argues, forgiving, as in remitting the consequences of the offence and moving forward, bears the risk of annulling its productive potential for future ethical deliberation (Vetlesen, 2014). The pains of remembrance are sometimes what keep us from repeating the sins of our forebears—or our own ones from the past. And, although "we might think that we are through with the past", as the philosopher Simon Critchley (2020) reminds us, the past is not always through with us (p. 3).

"Too late" are two sad words. Encountering them is like facing the limits of language. For what more can be said when it is too late? Sometimes, in therapy, words are whispering themselves toward truth, to existence. Forgiveness is a concept contained in a dictionary of unspoken words. It moves at a pace beyond time. Wittgenstein implored: "Whereof one cannot speak, thereof one must be silent." What happens when one can only forgive the forgivable? When too late, forgiveness can stir, but perhaps not mend, the unforgivable, the extreme. As when encountering death, or unbearable pain. Is forgiveness a paradox, a dream? It is a profound question, like a tide that strikes a cliff.

References

Ahmed, S. (2014). *The cultural politics of emotion* (2nd ed.). Edinburgh University Press.

Äikäs, T., & Fonneland, T. (2021). Animals in Saami shamanism: Power animals, symbols of art, and offerings. *Religions, 12*(4), 256. https://doi.org/10.3390/rel12040256

Arendt, H. (2018). *The human condition* (2nd ed.). University of Chicago Press.

Biesta, G. (2020). Can the prevailing description of educational reality be considered complete? On the Parks-Eichmann paradox, spooky action at a distance and a missing dimension in the theory of education. *Policy Futures in Education, 18*(8), 1011–1025. https://doi.org/10.1177/1478210320910312

Boekhoven, J. W. (2013). Public individualism in contemporary Dutch Shamanism. In W. Hofstee & A. van der Kooij (Eds.), *Religion beyond its private role in modern society* (pp. 245–257). Brill.

Critchley, S. (2020). *Tragedy, the Greeks and us*. Profile Books.

Derrida, J. (2001). *On cosmopolitanism and forgiveness* (Trans. M. Dooley & M. Hughes). Routledge.

De Waal, F. B. M., & van Roosmalen, A. (1979). Reconciliation and consolation among chimpanzees. *Behavioral Ecology and Sociobiology, 5*(1), 55–66. https://doi.org/10.1007/BF00302695

Harner, M. (1980). *The way of the shaman: A guide to power and healing*. Harper & Row.

Verbin, N. (2010). What is forgiveness? In M. R. Maamri, N. Verbin, & E. L. Worthington Jr. (Eds.), *A journey through forgiveness*. Inter-Disciplinary Press.

Vetlesen, A. J. (2007). *Hva er etikk? [What is ethics?]*. Universitetsforlaget.

Vetlesen, A. J. (2014). *Studier i ondskap [Studies in evil]*. Universitetsforlaget.

5

Longing, and Longing for Oneself: What Can Therapists Learn from "Soul Activism"?

Tone Grøver

Introduction

As a psychotherapist and a couples and family therapist, I encounter longing in many guises. It can be a matter of longing for concrete things, of existential themes, or it can be about a deep longing for something one can't quite identify where only the longing itself is certain. The allies of longing may be agitation, restlessness or a general dissatisfaction with life where the person feels that something needs to happen, something needs to be gained or something needs to change, before life is as it should be.

One of the forms of longing which I often encounter is the longing for oneself. It is often expressed with the sentence: "I have lost myself". My experience is that no kind of longing is filled with more despair than the longing for oneself. Behind it lies a wish for "coming home to myself". And often this expression follows: "I can't find myself". What is this

T. Grøver (✉)
Department of Family Therapy and Systemic Practice, Faculty of Social Studies, VID Specialized University, Oslo, Norway
e-mail: tone.grover@vid.no

T. Grover et al. (eds.), *New Horizons in Systemic Practice with Adults*, Palgrave Texts in Counselling and Psychotherapy, https://doi.org/10.1007/978-3-031-30526-9_5

phenomenon? Which selves are we longing for? Which self is lost? What can an exploration of the self teach us about what therapy might or should not contain when it comes to this painful longing for oneself? A premise for the longing for oneself is that a self exists as a kind of entity separate from other entities.

I got an opportunity to get closer to these questions when I had an encounter with former drug addicts who are running a mountain hotel and yoga retreat at Nøsen in Valdres, Norway. Amongst others, I got to know May-Rita Sætervoll and her way of thinking about longing and how to deal with it. It brought to me some critical reflections on therapy in our time. One such reflection is that therapy—also systemic therapy—in many ways has the separate self as a premise. The notion that there is a separate self is deeply rooted in our Western culture and is the basis also for most therapeutic processes. It has become a question for me whether systemic therapy has also come to be too much concerned with the *relationship between* separate selves, based on a fundamental assumption that the separate self exists. What could happen with therapy if the subject—the ego—is considered an illusion? I was inspired to explore this after a thought-provoking meeting with May-Rita and other ex-addicts.

During this exploration, I re-read Gregory Bateson's theories about the self and the ecology of the mental and became aware of how we—in systemic therapy—might have abandoned the most important point in his way of seeing the separate self as an illusion. Bateson had a gloomy view of a future where the human being would see itself as something other than, and separate from, nature (1972). Perhaps the separate self's longing for satisfaction is at the heart of the world's great problems at the same time as offering a key to understanding what we are longing for when we long for ourselves. If so, how does it affect the ethics of what we do in therapy and how we shape our roles as therapists?

The So-Called Self

In a systemic perspective, we see the self as relationally conditioned. A consequence of this is that the self is undergoing continuous change. However, in Bateson's work towards an understanding of the ecology of the mental, the self will not be found. And this is central to Bateson. He says that language, where the word "I" is most frequently used, makes us believe that the self is concrete and substantial. And with such a concreteness, the "self" has become a basis for much of psychology, psychiatry, sociology, economics, political science and so on, as well as being a fundamental premise in our language, culture and in daily thinking. And here a sort of misconnection occurs. We assume a premise, which leads to major consequences for us. Bateson saw the premise of the separate self as a big threat—and maybe the biggest threat—in our time. A threat not only to humans but to the entire Ecosystem.

Bateson instead sees the "self" as identical to and without separation from existence understood as Nature. To Bateson, Nature is a "system of consciousness" or "system of thinking", and in the ecological exchange it may be imperative that the human being learns—or rather, does not unlearn—thinking and being *as* Nature. He, therefore, speaks of the "so-called self" (1972). After the thought-provoking encounter with former addicts in the winter of 2021, I've been inspired to revisit this central aspect of Bateson's theories and ask what it may mean for therapy in our time. I have been inspired to ask whether a longing for oneself is a longing far outside of the identity and sense of self we so easily attribute to people, or to processes between people. Have we ended up reducing systemic understanding to the same thing as relational understanding, thereby losing something essential along the way?

Turning the Gaze Away from Oneself

It's the winter of 2021, and for ten days I lived close to a group of former drug addicts, some of them ex-convicts. They contribute as volunteers to the running of Nøsen Mountain Hotel and Yoga Retreat. I arrived there as a guest, during the off-season, to work on this chapter. As it turned out, I was the only guest for the first week. I told them that I was working on a chapter about longing. What did they think about that? It turned out that I had arrived at a treasure trove of longing. The craving for intoxication, they said, is precisely a form of longing. A longing for gaining contact with oneself, or for an escape from oneself and the pain of existence. It is a longing away from something, and towards something.

From restlessness towards calm. From turmoil towards peace. From boredom towards life. From pain towards rest. And the intoxication grants precisely the acute and short-lived dampening of longing. In this way, the intoxication is not itself the problem but an aid towards something fundamentally important. "The drug brings down the stress factors, the survival instinct gets a break, it's me time", as May-Rita expressed it. When "me time" is over, the longing has acquired a new companion, as the intoxication itself also becomes a source of longing, and in the long term turns into destruction.

May-Rita is in her early 50s and has volunteered at the Mountain Hotel and Retreat for several years, eventually gaining employee status. The days begin with yoga, meditation and a writing session, when she lets the words flow onto the page uncensored. Then it is time for the morning meeting with all volunteers and employees, followed by a long and demanding workday. She has more than 30 years of drug addiction behind her, the last 10 on heroin. Still, the craving for heroin torments her. She says: "It doesn't happen by itself. I choose Buddhist philosophy and yoga-philosophy. Daily practice; think well, do well, speak well. You need to trust that life wishes you well. But you also understand that you have to do the work yourself. You have your task in life." Through the conversation with her, I think about my own therapy sessions and how the attention is directed towards the person who shows up for therapy, which also makes the person I am talking to turn their attention towards themselves, their history and their problems. May-Rita talks about the opposite. She talks about a gaze turned away from oneself. She talks about doing the work herself.

When I returned from my stay at the retreat, I received one of the texts she has written. It is titled "Devotion (Soul Activism)". I believe she sent me this text because she cares about my struggle to understand longing, and which self we are longing after. In the text, she writes:

> we must be vulnerable, brave, open to the unknown, which in this encounter, in this moment becomes that which I regard as greater than us. Greater because it takes us in a direction of development. Development of ourselves as human beings, as individuals. Individuals who tie ourselves together in a single community. One 'us'. One 'we'. In the Way of Devotion,

my responsibility is to actively pursue and facilitate joy. Through love. THE LOVE OF WHAT I HOLD IN HIGHER REGARD THAN MYSELF. Of you and me, which is us and we. OF THE POWER WE together possess. As a sculptor cuts away layers of material, we remove the disturbances between us. Until we are left with what is real and true. When we can be completely open. And I mean 100 percent open. That Way. That is the way I wish to walk. That is the way I wish to fight for. (Emphasis hers) (May-Rita K. Sætervoll, personal correspondence, 6.12.2021, translated from Norwegian)

What is striking about this text is the absence of individualism. She highlights the "we", a *single* "us". She emphasizes devotion and love, beyond that which is tied to relations between people, a force which represents a different form of love. What insight might this bring?

A Departure from Nature?

How we read and understand this little excerpt of her text will depend on the glasses through which we see the world. In systemic psychotherapy and in family therapy, the glasses have different lenses, amongst them social constructivism, post-structuralism, critical realism and the systemic understanding stemming from Bateson. Common to constructivism, post-structuralism and critical realism is—in a highly simplified view—the idea that it is the people who construct what we perceive as "reality".

There is an essential difference between these theoretical approaches and the systemic understanding represented here by Bateson's theories. Bateson's theories take as a starting point the communication processes of Nature, and what he would later call "the god Eco". Through an understanding of the communication processes in Nature, Bateson creates his complex theories of the character of communication, and of the different levels of Mind (1972). Mind can be described as an immanent system of thought or consciousness which unfolds in the same way in coral reefs, in trees, in animals, in things, as in people (1972). And the consciousness of the god Eco consists of great complexity on different levels, from our little mentalities as people to the consciousness which is immanent in everything—but which is not free from influence from our ideas and actions. The reason for invoking the idea of a "god" is, as I understand it, a matter of emphasizing the all-encompassing immanent aspect—it is not a god in the sense which is familiar to us in the context of Western religion.

If we take as a starting point the complex systemic view as represented by Bateson, the object does not exist. Whenever we attempt to make an object out of something or someone, we have already departed from Nature's form of communication. An example used by Bateson was that of the pollution of a lake. When we pollute a lake, we are also polluting ourselves, physically and mentally. The lake does not exist as an object to be used by people. Yet it is not an ecological exchange of energy or physical substance which concerns Bateson, but the communicative exchange (1972). It is unfamiliar to us to relate to Nature as thinking or possessing some form of consciousness. But this is at the core of Bateson's theoretical work. He warned against seeing the human being as removed from the communicative ecology of Nature. He warned of the ecological catastrophe this would bring about. If one takes this ecology seriously, there are no aspects of life where it does not play out. The therapy room is no exception to this. Have our therapeutic forms of understanding, including systemic therapy, somehow departed from this? If the object does not exist, the subject cannot exist either. If the object does not exist, the subject is transcended—and we are in a non-dual understanding. If we hold on to this way of understanding humans, the "I" does not exist as anything else than a universal, everlasting process, with no birth and no death.

Today, publicly directed therapy is surrounded by goals, results, manuals, evidence-based methods and clearly structured packages. There is also an increasing despair connected to precisely this in many therapeutic circles where therapists experience an expectation of being "therapy machines". Why it has ended up this way is itself a complex sociological question, beyond the scope of this chapter. However, if we were to think as Nature, there would be no goals, no results, no efficiency, no methods, no solutions, no manuals in therapy. If we should stick to this form of communication, the self would not exist as a convergence point, not as a place, not as an entity to long after. In our time, is there something to be said for the revival of Bateson's ecological understanding in therapy? Can the longing for "oneself" be understood also in light of the global disasters we are faced with, and perhaps play a part in understanding the driving force behind what has led us towards the edge of the cliff? Because the longing for the self will involve an ongoing attempt to grasp something which can satisfy the separate self? Whereas, it is the opposite that can bring peace: a dissolution of the self, a belonging to existence itself? In a book about systemic therapy titled *New Horizon* (2023), while we know that the planet's ecology is seriously threatened, I believe these questions should be raised.

In a micro-context we may read May-Rita's text and ask: Is she contributing to the understanding of longing—and of longing for oneself—in a way that falls within Bateson's complex ecological understanding? Is it a contribution to understanding therapy, not as something separate, but as something which can be unified with the consciousness of Nature? If so, what will the consequences be for therapy?

Healing Through Surrendering

It is worth listening to and learning from people who accomplish one of the most difficult tasks we know—quitting heroin.

> Suffering through heroin withdrawal can't be explained with words. It is pure hell. I would rather chop off an arm than experience that. (Frank, quoted from Bu, 2016)

May-Rita managed it without therapy, without pharmaceutical assistance or what we call "treatment". And many of her fellow volunteers at Nøsen also managed it. How?

Here we should include some facts: The hotel, run by Alexander Medin, is behind two projects: "Back in the Ring" and "Gangster Yoga". "Back in the Ring" is a project for alcohol and drug addicts, based on Yoga philosophy: Yoga is practised to increase concentration and clear the mind, build down one's own ego and do good towards others. Today the project is in operation at 25 locations in Norway, and because it has proven to be helpful to drug addicts, it is now supported financially by the government. We should note the percentage of the participants that remain drug- and alcohol-free. It is, on average, 50–60%. Of those who complete the whole programme, nearly 100% become and remain completely drug-free. This is a percentage which is hardly seen elsewhere. What could this tell us?

The quotes from May-Rita, as well as accounts from other volunteers at Nøsen, point to something which they themselves view as important: turning the attention away from oneself and doing something for others. Seeing oneself as small in a greater context. Seeing meaning in what has happened; all the rough years May-Rita experienced, in an intoxicated state which shrouds the memory. In our conversation she says: "In retrospect, I see that everything has led me to where I am now". Through such a statement she highlights the trust she expresses towards existence; "trust that existence wishes me well". Herein lies the devotion she holds on to. And perhaps we can understand her expression, "soul activism", in this way. It is not about taking control, which is what we often associate with quitting drugs; not about seeking solutions, as we often do when problems arise; it is about the opposite: surrendering, and letting go of any concrete or separate self, and of control over life.

I often speak with people who feel that they have wasted a lot of life. For instance, through years of battling an eating disorder which has completely consumed their existence. When the disorder eventually loosens its grip, it is often succeeded by sorrow and despair over lost years, which becomes a new problem in itself. The person may blame themselves for failing to be healthier and more in control of life. May-Rita's more than 30 years of drug abuse comprise a large part of her life. Still, she sees them as forming the road that led her to where she is now, where she is grateful to be. Bateson said himself that he had never made a free choice. This may sound unfree, but is it? Can freedom be found precisely in surrendering to existence itself? It can be difficult for the human being not to see itself as in charge of matters, and this is where we have a misconnection, as Bateson suggests—in that we see the human being as outside of everything else. Then the belief in control comes naturally. This is what the historian Harari gloomily thematizes in *Homo Deus* (2017). In the study of Alcoholics Anonymous this is central to

Bateson: "The man against the bottle" won't help, it is the opposite the alcoholic needs: to surrender to a deeper belonging, away from the rational logic that has conquered the drug addict. In AA this is what they do, in such a way that they also surrender their identity and dedicate themselves to helping other alcoholics (1972).

His study of AA and the principles there can be recognized at Nøsen, although there is no known connection here. Let's see if we can take this further, in the understanding of the encounter with the longing for the self, and what this may mean for therapy.

Therapy: A Healing Process for the Therapist?

I see the contrast between what is happening in "Back in the Ring" and the therapy room. During a psychotherapy process, my attention is directed towards the person seeking therapy. The attention will, in the systemic spirit, strive towards being loving, accommodating, curious, unprejudiced, coequal and alternating between the light-hearted and the serious; all according to what the atmosphere allows. I will be attentive to my own resonance, and at times be transparent about this. This is how we as therapists have learned to be, and it feels right in every way. Yet, when faced with former addicts and ex-convicts at Nøsen, the following possibility occurs to me, and it may be a brazen thought: What if it is the therapist who undergoes the most important process in the therapy room? What if it is the therapist who, through the privilege of turning towards another, and being important to another, is actually the one who benefits the most? What if a therapeutic process can lead to a feeling of loneliness for the client because it is supposed to be about them—so that they can be more at ease with themselves? What would happen if we interchanged the roles? What would happen if the client turned to the therapist in empathetic curiosity and tried to discover what was troubling the therapist? (And something is in fact troubling the therapist in their life, don't worry about that.)

This is just a playful thought experiment, but it might cause us some constructive disturbance along the way. And this game has been played before, with roots in actual history: This is a part of the plot in Irvin

Yalom's historical novel about the relationship between Dr Josef Breuer (Freud's mentor) and the philosopher Friedrich Nietzsche (*When Nietzsche Wept*, 2012). While Breuer is supposed to be helping Nietzsche with his migraine attacks, their roles are gradually reversed, and Nietzsche ends up aiding Breuer with his deep existential anguish. In the process, Nietzsche's health improves, and the migraine attacks gradually subside. To begin with, this is a ruse on Dr Breuer's part. He intends to make himself into a project for Nietzsche in order to coax the resistant Nietzsche into agreeing to receive treatment. Behind the scenes there lurks a woman with whom Breuer has been infatuated, whom he wishes to impress and who was, in fact, Nietzsche's true love—but who had dumped him, still with a hope that Nietzsche would get help from Breuer. Through the process, Breuer gains Nietzsche's attention and help to explore his existential issues, which is a great benefit to both Breuer and Nietzsche. Eventually, it ends as it inevitably must; Breuer's plot comes to light, and they resolve the potential break between themselves with perfect transparency. And the transparency is healing for them both. In this way, the roles of client and therapist are broken, resulting in a healing community. In May-Rita's text, this is denoted as 100% openness. "Until we are left with what is real and true".

When I receive a family in therapy where the father, the mother or both express great worry about their adolescent child, and the concern for the child is what brings them to me, it sometimes happens, if the climate, atmosphere and contact are right, that I turn to the child and ask: "What's wrong with your parents? Are they this worried all the time?" Not rarely, this sparks delight in the young one. She and I are now on the same team, and we are removed from the therapeutic discourse; we are a little shaken in our understanding of the context. But not only that; the parents can—in a humorous setting—feel the effects of being made an object, and of the power games of the therapy room. For a moment they become an object for the others to view—the problem object—and they get to taste the effects of this.

At Nøsen the participants are in a context where they, through yoga-philosophy (which means unity/binding together), don't have the person as an object in their framework of understanding. Nor do they seek to be subjects side by side. In yoga philosophy, as well as in Buddhism, there is interbeing, where subjects and objects are abolished in the name of nonduality. This is fundamental to the philosophy of the place. Buddhism, which is important to May-Rita, underlines the significance of transparency, in order to avoid positions of power. I see many parallels to Bateson's postulate about thinking as Nature. I also see why Bateson was curious about Buddhism (although he refused to be categorized as a Buddhist), and Buddhists about him (Parks, 2019). And for me, it becomes exciting to ask again, whether we might come to hold on too tightly to the self as a subject, or object, in therapy, even though we are systemically anchored. And that the very act of helping might tighten our grip around a false premise about a separate self. And if we are to avoid this, how are we to orient ourselves?

If we follow the thought experiment above, it is possible to say that the therapist should be just as enriched in the therapy process as the so-called client. And that it is perhaps a signal that interbeing and a nourishing community has been abandoned, in favour of a subject–object relationship, if the therapist becomes tired and fatigued. And perhaps there is a discourse to be had as to whether we, as so-called helpers, are there for clients, while the clients are not there for us. If we get tired, is it perhaps a signal that we are giving ourselves an elevated status? With the risk of holding the person we talk to, in the therapy room, firmly as an object, with the damage that can bring. Is it a question? A similar question is raised by Sheehan and Vetere in their chapter (this volume) where they describe the experience of love understood as *agape* (Sheehan & Vetere, 2023).

Love as a Transaction or as a Universal Dimension? Soul Activism

What May-Rita does, as I understand her, is to connect to a community where she can mean something to others, and others can mean something to her. Of staying at Nøsen, she says: "Being here is a longing for a harmonious symphony". It is the harmonious that becomes her orientation. In it, she does not seek loving relationships to satisfy her needs: Love is something she is and wishes to be and connect to. This is what she is referring to when she talks about "love as something greater than myself", as I understand her from our conversations.

Nature's way of thinking could well be understood as "symphony", in the sense that it is an everlasting interplay, a never-ending exchange, which seeks to maintain a balance; what Bateson called homeostasis. When Nature today is answering us in the way it currently is, with droughts, floods, avalanches and so on, it is not to punish mankind but to regain a point of balance. Biologists and climate scientists all over the world agree that Nature will eventually succeed in this. It is patient, and it will take as long as it needs—perhaps a million years. Nature's current response is, so to speak, a more dramatic part of the symphony which it is always playing. Bateson has been criticized for refraining from tackling the power games we clearly see in human relations—in organizations, between countries, in all kinds of contexts—of course in the therapy room as well. Yes, power games are what constitute the world of humans, if we are to take Foucault seriously: "There are only mutual relations, and the constant divides in intention, in relation to each other" (translated from Foucault in Heede, 2004, p. 14). When Bateson wasn't so preoccupied with power and power games, it was perhaps precisely because of his orientation towards the ecology of the mental, and towards Nature's way of thinking.

When May-Rita expresses her trust that "existence wishes me well", it promotes in her a calmness, a sense of love greater than that which plays out in the transaction of a relationship. In contrast to our usual thought of giving and receiving love—the road is short to thinking that "I" or a "self" finds the greatest peace and safety when it disappears as an ego, becoming unified with something "higher than myself". Is there a deep desire in the human being to dissolve as a separate being? As in the famous painting of Edvard Munch *the kiss*. It depicts two people kissing, although they share a single face, *fallen* into love. But when another person is what you try to dissolve into, problems arise, as we know.

I would think many therapists share the following experience with me: When we work with a couple or a family on difficulties in their relationships, we might end up "moving furniture around", with the result being a different kind of mess than we started with. Someone else ends up as the injured party. Was it a departure from love as a transaction that Bateson meant when discussing the meaning of love and of loving: "I'm willing to love animals, ships, and all sorts of quite inappropriate objects. Even, I suppose, a computer, if I had the care for one, because care and maintenance are in this picture too" (quoted in Ølgaard, 2001, pp. 246–247).

Much of the couples and family relations I encounter in my work are about love as a transaction. And the transactions are connected to separate selves' longing. This makes us vulnerable and dependent. Precisely the dependence on the other's way of being is a recurring theme in couples therapy. Are we playing along with this in systemic therapy?

After the conversation with May-Rita, I had a few therapy sessions with a mother who had lost contact with her adult daughter. The daughter had broken contact with the mother and they hadn't seen each other in years. Naturally, this engendered difficult emotions in the mother: She struggles to understand, finds the daughter cold and selfish, and can't see why it has turned out this way. She suspects her ex-husband of being behind it all, pulling strings and creating animosity. But she nevertheless feels hurt by her daughter. She is unsure of whether she will be able to forgive her daughter should she turn to her mother for support at some point in the future. There seems to be too much bitterness and pain in the way. This is very understandable. Her longing creates pain, not contact or reconciliation. With May-Rita in the back of my mind, I asked her: Do you think it is possible for you to ground yourself in love for your daughter without getting anything but rejection in return? If I suggest that love does not have to be an exchange, but rather something you can be, something you can represent and rest in, independently of your daughter's choices—what would this lead to? The mother's answer was that this surprisingly helped her find calmness within. What the mother and I are doing is, perhaps, to leave the transactional understanding of love, which is in turn based on the idea of separate, concrete "selves". Such ideas tend to engulf couples and families in their struggle to find their way, which makes so many of us feel contingent on how we are received by others. What the mother and I do together is to see her striving as pure love gone astray.

A woman I work with has struggled with her recurring depression. She had a parallel individual therapy process for her depression at another place where she was encouraged to go home to her husband and tell him that she needed him to give her the confirmation she longed for. She felt so miserable in the lack of confirmation, and even more miserable for being the cause of the spouse's despair and loneliness, in the shadow of her depression. She constantly saw him unhappy. All her life, she had been struggling with the feeling of not being valuable. The depression made this feeling grow. Now she was encouraged to stand up for herself, asking him for confirmation. The husband, feeling so lonely because of her depression, became completely locked. "I can't", he said. "So sorry, it's just not possible any longer. It will be fake, we have no true contact. I'm so sorry". His face was loaded with pain. I asked the wife what this appealed to in her. "I want to give him a hug, I want to comfort him", she replied. "So why not do it right now?" I asked. She put her arm around her husband, and he cried for the first time in years. He said: "You must understand that I miss you". "How is it for you to hear that he misses you?" I asked. In a strong voice, she said: "It's wonderful". The interplay of her looking at her inadequacy, and feeling guilty for her depression, turned upside down at that moment. Her status of being "The problem" disappeared, for the here and now.

Perhaps the radically different understanding that the self does not exist as anything other than part of a communication process, and a radically different understanding of what love is, is what can sometimes bring the longing—and the accompanying pain—to an end. Could this move us away from the idea of *accomplishing* something in therapy, towards accepting and living with the fact that others are how they are? This does not mean accepting any and all behaviour from others, but being a better influence on others, and ourselves, through trust and seeing ourselves as representing a "higher" love. As we experience Nature, we recognize that the ecological processes are all about non-selfishness, every process is there for the process itself. Such insight finds further echoes in the Sheehan and Vetere chapter (this volume) on *agape* love.

I believe this "higher love" is what May-Rita calls "soul activism". Activism for a more peaceful existence—a "symphony". It is an understanding of "soul", which is not so dependent on a relational game with love as a "commodity", to gain or to lose, and therefore more secure. It is an understanding of "soul" that is reminiscent of Bateson's understanding of the immanent consciousness—which he feared could be knocked off balance if we were to disconnect from it and cease to think as it. Then Nature will begin a healing process, which "may be ruthless. Whole species may be exterminated in the process" (1979, p. 206). Is this where we are? If so, should we care—as therapists and professionals?

Are We All Therapists?

I think the questions above should be opened, not answered. But I wonder if our time—with uncertainty on so many levels, not least uncertainty about our future existence on Earth—demands we ask? Are we holding on to a logic that permeates human actions on earth and that potentially destroys the same world? And does therapy lean on this same logic?

There is an enormous power in the therapeutic discourse. By education, therapists as a group are supposed to know what illness is, what problems are and what treatment is. And we prescribe our own medicine, which also depends on us. This all relies on the premise that we as therapists are subjects, knowing something about objects. Looking back, it is surprising to see how methods and approaches in therapy turned out to be so far removed from "Nature's way of thinking" in the wake of Bateson and ended up as tactical, strategic, structural, paradoxical, intervening, narrative and so on. All ways of *accomplishing* something. Perhaps Bateson's theories of Mind are too far from our instrumentally rational reality and our need for accomplishing something as therapists. Our need to be valued as therapists.

May-Rita represents a way of life, and a view of life, which can be understood as a dissolution of the individual, separate self; as a stepping away from love as a transaction and resting in a "greater" form of love. In meeting with her and her way of quitting drugs, a therapist's role must dissolve. She would be as much therapist for the therapist, as the other way around. If a therapist insisted on the role, and if she had bowed to it, we can clearly see it could have been in the way of healing. Her experiences can inspire us to revive Bateson's understanding of the immanent consciousness which permeates and unfolds in everything, and the ecological understanding of life—what May-Rita calls "soul activism". And her experience can also inspire us to ask how therapy can step out of all power games based on subject–object and subject–subject understanding, because the power games themselves are destructive for healing, no matter how subtle they are. Might we, as therapists, stand in the way of healing, if we are not willing to see ourselves as nothing but part of a nourishing community?

If so, the question becomes: What do I *do* as a therapist in therapy? If we are to learn from May-Rita and other volunteers at Nøsen, we can say that we're all patients, we're all clients, and we're all therapists. They inspire us to go deeper into systemic ethics and challenge ourselves in the role we possess. Are we sufficiently open to the creativity which may arise if we lean into the nourishing community rather than the roles of the client and therapist? Are we as therapists sufficiently open to that undressing of ourselves as not knowing? And one might wonder if the many evaluations, manuals and methods that have found their way into therapy bring about a climate that hinders nourishing communities.

We can't easily change basic premises, demands, goals, results, methods, manuals, efficiency and throughput. The premises are here, and they are not all for the bad. Some of the justification is to ensure that as many as possible get the help they ask for and many are helped as well. The worry is that we allow the premises to dominate so much, also where they are pushing the self towards more felt isolation. What could we, based on "Nature's way of thinking", be and do in our roles, given the rational premises?

Given my reasoning in this chapter, and what I've learned from May-Rita and the volunteers at Nøsen, we should be curious about what opens up to us if we disconnect from thoughts of methods and professional approaches and exchange the idea of therapy and therapy room for the idea of a nourishing community and a room for collaboration. Over the course of the 20 years I have spent as a therapist, one fashionable method after another has come and gone. They are introduced with the same enthusiasm every time, accompanied by percentagewise success rates and fade away just as predictably. If we learn from May-Rita and volunteers at Nøsen, we turn our attention away from the methods and roles, towards the nourishing community. Towards the symphony. Even in cases where external pressure is mounting and conditions are tight. This idea is in principle not very different from the creative forms of therapy we know in social constructionism and collaborative practice, with inspiration from, among others, Kenneth Gergen and Harlene Anderson. Nor is it far from key elements in Deliberate Practice, a new and growing branch of therapist training, that abandons methods and models and goes straight to training and feedback on practice in the here and now (Bate et al., 2022, Rousmaniere, 2016). The difference is that the point of orientation suggested here is not social, human construction, but identification with Nature. It requires a way of listening to Nature, and to oneself as a piece of Nature, which we may have to rediscover in ourselves as therapists to be able to help others rediscover themselves the same way. It also requires understanding that the longing for oneself can be a deep longing to belong to a universal kind of love. The forms of yoga, meditation, love and silence, which allow listening to and dissolving into existence, can become a main source of inspiration for therapists.

A nourishing community is constituted by mutual dependence, like the fruit needs the bumblebee, and vice versa. Is it possible to have such a community, which lasts for 45–60 minutes at a time over a few sessions—as is the premise for much of therapy? Let us again derive inspiration from Irvin Yalom. In his latest book, *A Matter of Death and Life* (2021), which he wrote together with his now deceased wife Marilyn, he talks about the last patient he is seeing. Yalom is burdened by his wife's fight with cancer, and his memory is suffering. He is in his late 80s. He has forgotten that his patient is supposed to come, and he has forgotten the e-mail she sent him. She doesn't take it well and feels invisible and insignificant. Yalom explains that it is not about her. He tells her of his failing memory and of his wife of 65 years, who is so ill, and how badly she suffers. He apologizes deeply for allowing this to affect her. The following day he also writes her an e-mail, apologizing again. In the reply she sends him, she tells him that of all they have done together over the course of the therapy sessions, his opening up to her is the most important. She says that suddenly, they were no longer patient and therapist, they were human beings together. And this made a deep impression on her. They were stripped of roles, power and the "game" of therapy. For her, this effect lived on. And for him, her letter was a relief.

With all this said: of course, those (often young people) who are training to become therapists may need something to hold on to. We have all needed this. But should young therapists learn methods and approaches with the clear understanding that all methods have the capacity to work against their purpose and that they, as soon as they are confident enough, should dare to emerge more as a human being, without a method to hide behind? And if methods are in play, we should be totally transparent about it, inviting the clients to decide whether it works well, or not, in the interplay. This chapter points in that direction.

I suggest that we continue exploring what a self is (or rather isn't) and how we can form nourishing communities with the greatest possible degree of transparency. Where the longing is turned away from the ego's satisfaction to a dissolving of self, into interbeing. Maybe we need to lean more towards Nature's inherent wisdom, not only to shape more true meetings in therapy but to be able to live in harmony and contact with our Ecosystem and life on earth.

References

Bate, J., Prout, T. A., Rousmaniere, T., & Vaz, A. (2022). *Deliberate practice in child and adolescent psychotherapy*. American Psychological Association.

Bateson, G. (1972). *Steps to an ecology of mind*. Chandler Publishing Company.

Bateson, G. (1979). *Mind and nature. A necessary unity*. Dutton.

Bu, Kari and Dimitri. (2016, 21. oktober). Erlikselgere forteller hvordan rusen virker = *Oslo*. https://www.erlik.no/erlik-selgere-forteller-hvordan-rusen-virker/ [Islike sellers tell how the drug works].

Harari, Y. N. (2017). *Homo Deus*. SD Books.

Heede, D. (2004). *Det tomme menneske. Introduktion til Michel Foucault [The empty man. Introduction to Michel Foucault]*. Museum Tusculanum Press.

Ølgaard, B. (2001). *Kommunikation og økomentale systemer i følge Gregeory Bateson [Communication and eco mental systems accordingly to Gregory Bateson]*. Akademisk forlag.

Parks, T. (2019). *Impossible choices.* https://aeon.co/essays/gregory-bateson-changed-the-way-we-think-about-changing-ourselves

Rousmaniere, T. (2016). *Deliberate practice for psychotherapists.* Routledge.

Sheehan, J., & Vetere, A. (2023). The therapeutic relationship: A systemic view of Agape. In *New horizons for systemic practice with adults and families.* Palgrave.

Yalom, I. D. (2012). *When Nietzsche wept.* Harper Perennial.

Yalom, I. D., & Yalom, M. (2021). *A matter of death and life.* SD Books.

6

Giving Resonance and Room to Spirituality in Systemic Practice

Åse Holmberg and Bengt Karlsson

Introduction

To be human is to be spiritual. The spirit, which comes from the word "breath", is our vital essence, the power of life. The spiritual force is important for living a meaningful life for ourselves and others in a global and diverse world. For many, the spiritual life is a natural part of their lives; for others, it is more non-conscious and unreflective.

In our time, we see increasing attention to spiritual perspectives. The world is characterized by progress, consumption and quick fixes. There are also a lot of challenges in our time which can create unrest, such as the war in Europe, environmental disturbances, increasing poverty and social and economic differences between people and countries. More and more

Å. Holmberg (✉)
VID Specialized University, Oslo, Norway
e-mail: ase.holmberg@vid.no

B. Karlsson
University of South-Eastern Norway, Drammen, Norway

© The Author(s), under exclusive license to Springer Nature Switzerland AG 2023   **81**
T. Grover et al. (eds.), *New Horizons in Systemic Practice with Adults*, Palgrave Texts in
Counselling and Psychotherapy, https://doi.org/10.1007/978-3-031-30526-9_6

people are suffering from mental disorders, and many feel lonely and outside society. Ontological questions emerge. Who am I and whom do I want to be? How do I find meaning and coherence in our time? Although many people in our society are materially well off, there seems to be a longing for something more, something bigger and something deeper that science cannot give.

This chapter will focus on the spiritual human and show how spiritual perspectives are strongly linked to systemic practices. We will take a closer look at the concept of spirituality, and link it to spiritual perspectives like love, wonder and complexity. We will include some voices from an ongoing study about young adults' experiences and reflections on the spiritual life, and we reflect on the need for therapists to find their spiritual path. The question is how systemic professionals can provide resonance and space in their practice for clients' spiritual reflections and experiences. The theme has until now had limited attention in the systemic family therapy field, and there is little research (Holmberg, 2018).

Our Journeys

Åse

I grew up in Norway at the end of the 1960s in a Protestant family where the importance was to go to church, read the Bible and live as dutifully as possible. It was important to be active, and therefore I became a leader early on. However, I have been critically reflective for as long as I can remember, and it has been difficult for me to accept established truths. I believe that the spiritual and God are always greater than humans can understand. My experience is that there can be a lack of space in the church, and it can be difficult to be touched and find nourishment for the soul.

Anyway, the spiritual part of life is a mystery and I believe there is more to discover. I have surrendered a dualistic image of God, and hold that God loves his creation and wants contact. Life is deeply meaningful, and one's existence has a purpose. I think our most important task in the world is to carry on the love of God. The only thing we know is now—and now matters. The spirituality of humans can make a difference in relation to self, others, nature and life in general.

Bengt

I grew up in a family different from Åse. My parents were members of the Labour party and religion was based on Marx's thesis: "Religion is opium for the people". Although I was baptized, and we were always in the church for Christmas, I refused to have any form of confirmation as a teenager. I was politically active in a left-wing party until I was 35 years old. Questions concerning the meaning of life, whether there is a life after death, what is humanity, what is to believe or not to believe and what is there to believe in, have always interested me. To me, these are different aspects of spirituality. Whenever and wherever I am, I often visit a church or a chapel. When I am in these rooms, I often feel humble, mindful and open. I have a strong bodily awareness of being on holy ground. I think of this as spirituality in my life. I do not know what it is. I know how it feels in my mind and my body.

The Spiritual Human

We are all on a spiritual journey. Originally, spirituality comes from the word "spirit", which in Greek (anemos) means "breath" and can be seen as human beings' vital essence or life force. Human spirituality is part of an ecological or holistic view, our ontology, and influences physical, psychological and social life. This power of life is closely connected to existential perspectives like meaning, values, hope and faith, and helps people to find connection and direction in life. This is not a static condition, but a process that changes and develops throughout life. The spirituality of humans has different sources, depending on the human view of life. Everyone has their unique spiritual journey developed through life from birth to death, which acts as an important contributor to human satisfaction and growth in life (Miller & Thoresen, 2003).

Spirituality is a word that includes many perspectives and can be difficult to put into words. It can be words like the philosophy of life, religion, faith, meaning, existential perspectives, view of reality, soul, the sacred, ethics—and spirituality.

To be spiritual is a universal human dimension, but people can reflect on this in varying degrees throughout life. In some periods the spiritual life will probably be stronger, perhaps when one is at a crossroads, in crisis, transitions, or in case of illness and death. The spirituality of life is connected to culture, history and relations, and each one shapes spirituality from this. This creates the basis for the understanding and experiences of:

- Meaning—the ontological significance of life.
- Values—faith/philosophy/ideology of life, how we want to live our life.
- Transcendence—our relation to the non-material, what we do not fully understand. Something is greater than us, we are part of something bigger.
- Connections—relationships to others, God/Higher Power, nature. Our cohesion with the abstract and absolute in life, death and our existence.
(Serander, 2018; Swinton, 2001)

Spirituality seems to be something we exercise and experience, like a way of being about self, others, culture, nature and life and includes a transcendent dimension. The invisible world seems to be much larger than the visible world. The spirituality of humans is bodily and closely connected to emotions and feelings. The body holds meaning, culture, rationality and tradition. A close relationship exists between the mind and the body. People experience their world through the body, and the body also has a social influence on our surroundings. We have a bodily repertoire that we automatically express, consciously or unconsciously (Merleau-Ponty, 2002). Spiritual experiences often exist partly in the language but are felt fully in the body. The spiritual body can be an important source of knowledge. Recognition of clients' bodily experiences is therefore important.

Humans have several spiritual sources, like music, nature, churches, literature, holy scripters and relations. Spirituality is about asking the big existential questions: Why am I here? What is life? How to create a more loving and connected world? You can read more about existential themes in couple therapy by Riste Andersen and Thiis-Evensen in this book.

Religious Life

Religion is an important source for many people and can be part of a human's spiritual life. Religion comes from the Latin word "Religare", which means "to connect, to bind", a bond between humanity or a power greater than human beings. Religion often refers to formal systems of belief and belonging to a religious group or community, usually including a God or a higher power. The various religions provide values and guidelines for life (Swinton, 2001; Walsh, 2009). Scientists and sociologists have prophesied the downfall of religion, but as the world has evolved, it has not lost its relevance. Many people need something to hold on to, something to lean on in storms, something bigger than themselves. The religious appeal lies in the idea that God or the Universe touches us. It is a practice of relationships. Praying, for example, is both listening and responding. Rosa (2019) calls it "deep resonance, there is one who hears you, who understands you, who can find ways and means of reaching you and responding to you" (p. 261). It is the promise that the universe of God still speaks even when we are incapable of hearing it. In every human soul, there is a glimpse of God. Most religions have an overarching idea of charity, reciprocity and justice built into their ethics and legal system. The "golden rule" is an example of that. However, there are also examples of religions that can block the spiritual world, which act oppressively and close human rights. If love is the most important element in religion, it has to create a universe of hope, nourishment and liberation for the human soul.

Humanistic Spirituality

In this chapter, we embrace a humanistic spirituality which goes beyond religion, which means we are not concerned with what separates us, but rather what unites us. We prefer a more cosmic we, where we look through a cosmic lens, where the love for oneself and others is the driving force. Love is a paradox and involves a clear decision, a flow of energy that is willingly exchanged and allowed without demanding payment in return. We often have limited constructions of spirituality and religion created by our culture, traditions and experiences, and acknowledge that spiritual wisdom is far greater than we can comprehend. Spiritual wisdom is more a synthesis than analysis, more paradoxical than linear, more a dance than a march. We prefer non-dualistic thinking with the ability to read the moment with a non-judgmental and non-exclusionary attitude. If there are parts we do not understand, we will leave things open— and let them speak to us (Rohr, 2014).

Voices of Spirituality from Youths

Before we move on to trying to link spirituality and systemic practice together, we will highlight some voices from an ongoing study of young adults about their experiences and reflections on spirituality. Learning from practice has always been an important perspective in systemic therapy, and these groups of youths can give us important perspectives.

Ten young people were interviewed, aged 20–32, born Norwegian, all unemployed and part of network groups organized by the Norwegian Labour and Welfare Administration in Norway. They live different lives and have various mental, physical and relational challenges, but all had wise and important stories to share about this topic. One important finding in the study is that despite a lot of difficulties, mostly all the youths were filled with love and care and longed to be something for others.

David, for example, who struggles with a meaningless and lonely life, refers to an African proverb that says: A child that is not embraced by the village will burn it down to feel its warmth. He continues: You need to find belonging, and shared meaning, you need to feel that you are part of something. One thing that makes me happy is animals, children and good company. I miss physical contact.

Several of the other young people also point to this; to be there for somebody is the ultimate meaning, I try to make others feel good, try to help, and, if I see someone having a hell of a time, I'm having a hell of a time myself.

Simon lost his dad when he was eight years old. Asking him what helped him after his father's death, he replies: "I become fonder of people, caring more about people. If they say they have no problems, then you need to follow up and see if they are fine".

Longing for Belonging

The youths say, As humans we are completely dependent on each other. We need each other to live good lives. For example, Simon says:

> Nature has its system that works. But everything is one thing. If it is something outside the thing, you are still part of that thing. So how do we destroy nature? By destroying yourself. We need each other to help us correct and learn from each other. After all, we are nature. And it is, in a way, perfect.

David has similar reflections:

> I've never had any affiliation…it's hard to produce. People need other people. It is a truth that no one can contradict. We all know it, on a completely genuine level. There is no place for me in society. Dad died when I was 16, and after that everything fell apart.

We also see despair among the youths. Elly and Louisa, two young women say:

> Society is in many ways so closed. You can go out and still feel trapped. Most people are very contained. Humans are very fond of thinking about themselves.
> Nobody listens to me. I am worthless. That's the feeling I'm left with. Why don't they listen to me? Am I that worthless? Do I have no dignity?

The Mystery of Life

The youths have many spiritual reflections about the mystery of life. They talk about God or the Universe, death, life before birth and after death, finding peace, dreams and meaning of life, supernatural experiences, meditation and the future.

David says:

Many of my problems are existential problems. And every time people ask me what I need to go ahead, I say; a crazy philosophy professor, that's what I need. I have tried to talk to doctors, therapists, or psychologists about such things, but they say that we don't talk about this because it is not interesting to them. But anyway, it is such things that occupy me, and talking could have helped me get some more stable footing in this existential world we live in.

Life is about living here and now. And that's my biggest problem, I don't live here and now. It's because I have problems on a completely different level. When I was young, I got stuck on a metaphysical mountain and never got back.

There is a lot of uncertainty among the youths related to these topics. Brian for example says he has a fear of death. He thinks a lot about death. If he is too much by himself and thinks about it, he can completely break down, start hyperventilating and have an anxiety attack. Much of the time they "turn off" their brain in order not to think about it. Brian says he goes out and parties a lot, but it is just to get rid of the bad thoughts.

Spirituality and Systemic Practice

Keeping these youths in mind, we will now take a look at how to connect systemic thinking and practice with spirituality. Systemic thinking is not a method or a technique, but a way to understand human difficulties. Problems and events are part of contexts and contribute to an expanded perspective on people and problems. Each one constructs his understanding of the world and how we communicate will therefore be decisive for well-being, growth and development.

Systemic therapy and thinking are based on philosophical and humanistic practice. Our self is not an individual identity, but we are part of an ecological community, where we have responsibility for each other. Bateson (2000) talked about an ecological sacred world, where the relationship is the smallest unit.

We think, to be systemic, is to naturally adopt a spiritual focus. Bateson (2000) encouraged us to look beyond and contemplate "the pattern" that connects. A systemic view of life is a holistic view of life, where also humans' spiritual life is part of the whole.

To Be Met in Love

In an ecological world, we all have a responsibility to each other. How we act and take care of each other means something. In systemic work, we invite collaboration, and we believe that people have resources and opportunities for change. It requires that clients are seen and met, in love.

As far as we can see, love seems to be the most important spiritual need. Love is a universal language, the attraction of all things towards all things. It is an underlying energy, so simple that it is difficult to learn it in words. But we know when we feel it. We also know when we feel the opposite—resistance and coolness. People will always remember how you make them feel. Love is the metaphysical foundation for everything. We long for union, and to love and be loved. Real love changes us in the depth and expands the spirit.

We are created in relationships. Therapy is a relational dialogical process where the relationship is crucial to the outcome. Deepest in ourselves and others we find love. Through listening, showing respect, tolerance, understanding and acceptance, we bring out the love in the other (Schibbye, 2009). "There is a crack in everything, there when the lights go in", Leonard Cohen says. Great love has the potential to open the heart space and then the mind space. In the chapter written by Sheehan and Vetere, "The Therapeutic Relationship: A Systemic View of Agape", they also explore the experience of love in therapy.

How to Be Familiar with the Unfamiliar?

As systemic therapists, we respond to uniqueness. No one is the same. We see each face of the other and try to meet everyone with respect. We do not want to rise above the other but give a hand that can give strength and freedom. This is an attitude, not a technique. Through the fact that I embrace and acknowledge the other's life, it can open the space for the client to reflect on me. This can be easy on the page, but quite more difficult in real life. It can be easy to acknowledge something we know, something we can do, and easier to express in positive terms. We think all religions and spiritual thinking must be treated with respect because it is the other's life. At the same time, we recognize that there is also spiritual and religious thinking that is unhealthy and depressing. We want a practice based on humanist values, human rights, and the laws of the country. It is our belief that everyone needs to be met in love.

Recognition is closely connected to the word "resonance". Looking at the concept, resonance is both a physical and a musical concept. The sociologist Hartmut Rosa says it is the moment when the world sings. Resonance is produced only when the vibration of one body stimulates the other to produce its frequency (Rosa, 2019, p. 165). Therefore, resonance is a kind of relationship with the world, formed through emotions and interests. It is not an echo, but a responsive relationship, where both sides speak with their voice but are also open enough to be affected or reached by each other. As humans, we are created for resonance. We need security, protection and care. That is what attachment theory has taught us. We know that our emotional and social development is affected by how we are met and received (Dallos & Vetere, 2022). We mutually create each other.

The ability for resonance is under pressure in our society. The pressure can lead to alienation, an exhaustion of the self, where relationships become instrumental. Seikkula (2008) says that a surprising number of professionals find it difficult to be in dialogue with clients and colleagues. Many professionals seem to be most concerned with being proficient in different methods and interventions, which can take the focus away from the simple thing of being present in the moment and letting all voices be heard. If resonance is part of the solution, it is initially about bringing oneself into play as an instrument in relational interactions (Tønder & Karlsson, 2020). In Vetere's chapter in this book, "Coming Full Circle with the Neuroscience", she writes more about trust and connection.

As systemic therapists, we bring with us our own experience and history, and this will probably have a great influence on what we choose to emphasize in the dialogue (Jensen, 2008). If spiritual perspectives are foreign to us, both personal and professional, there is a high probability that we do not give resonance to these dimensions of the clients' lives.

The therapist's values, interests and personal experiences will create a context for the therapeutic work. However, the ability to resonate and establish connections and responsive relationships can be trained and refined. As therapists, we need to ask ourselves if we are a door opener or a door closer to the client's spiritual room. Knowing there is room can make a difference for the client (Holmberg et al., 2017).

Making Room for Wondering and Reflections

The message from Bateson was to bring back the sacred (1987). Nature was his world of research, and he looked for interactions and connections. We do not have all the answers, and never will. Bateson called it a cybernetic spirituality, based on humility and endless curiosity. This allows for a both/and attitude, rather than an either/or attitude, where reflections are shaped as thoughts, ideas, and questions. We need to focus on what we believe is useful for the client (Andersen, 2011) Many clients feel an attraction to the spiritual and to the sacred. So how do we keep our senses open to this?

The not–knowing position is for many therapists a well-known perspective (Andersen, 1997). In therapy, every human is a new experience. We need to be sensitive to differences. Research and general knowledge are part of our profession, but it is not certain that this is suitable for those sitting in front of us. What is most useful for the clients? Working as systemic practitioners we try to be sensitive and ready to meet the differences, and what is new for you. In our world, this is also about being open to the spiritual universe of the clients. A creative therapist can explore what is new and different, and what can be of help and benefit to the individual.

Science and knowledge are not something static and ready-made that we discover. It is something we create in the face of reality. We cannot find everything in a textbook. We soon can find ourselves separate and without wonder. We have to participate in life itself. Not knowing is an exciting starting point for creativity and will hopefully make us more open-minded. And perhaps a better listener, too.

Embrace the Complexity

No one can overview a person's total complex situation. There is not one reality, but a multiverse where everyone has their understanding of reality. In a systemic world, we respect differences and know that no two situations or experiences are the same.

We have an innate ability to communicate and synchronize with others. Many religions are concerned with relationships and community. For example, in Christianity, God is a relationship. It is our belief that we are created in the image of God and thus created as relational. Thus, for us, all living things will have an imprint of a living God.

The beauty of creation confronts people with enigmatic depths, and it creates a wonder about how everything can be connected in a mysterious whole. It is quite fascinating that the cosmos can form a harmonious whole in its great diversity. Existence has an inherent structure and a given meaning. As humans, it can be difficult to reconcile ourselves with this whole. The experience shows that we create an imbalance in our greed and selfishness. Therefore, we have to live with nature and respect and learn about ecology and the natural balance. It has all we need—to know the divine, to know yourself, to know life, and even to trust death. Rohr (2014) says, by reading reality from inside this circle of creation, and with the eyes of nature, you will inherently know you are already in a sacred space, and you will know that you belong. As therapists, we believe this calls for humility, and will perhaps make us even more curious about what we do not yet know.

As systemic therapists, we prefer a non-dualistic worldview. Everything is connected, everything belongs to each other, and we are part of the circle of life, in dialogue. We will not separate mind, body and spirit, but rather explore how people's different perspectives affect each other in a relational context. We mutually create each other. The sacred can be seen in the wordless, in the sensing, in the trust, in the presence and in the meeting with a client. The sacred moves and touches us. It requires us to stop and be present in the now. A busy and hectic life can make us blind, deaf and strangers to the sacred (Martinsen, 2005).

The Therapist's Spiritual Path

Who we are as therapists means something. In meeting spiritual clients there is a need to increase personal awareness and competence and work with personal hindrances (Holmberg et al., 2021). We will here highlight two perspectives we find important: To connect with our inner life and give time for contemplation.

Earlier in our chapter, we could read about the importance of meeting clients in love. We think love is the most important of all our spiritual needs. Helping clients find their "flow", as therapists, we also need to take care of our hearts. To follow the heart is to have contact with what is living inside us. What gives me peace, love and meaning in my life? We need access to our feelings, so we are emotionally available. Developing spirituality is about expanding our capacity to love (Rohr, 2014). Life is not about me, I am all about life. We know that people live a better life without bitterness and anger. If people can change their hearts, is that what we call healing?

Time for Contemplation

If we will get in touch with our inner life, we believe we need time for contemplation. Many people have busy working days, and we can easily run from ourselves. Just take time to be quiet, find silence, breathe calmly and just listen. Some take a walk and just listen to nature. How do I find my path in life? What gives me meaning in life? Contemplation can help us look at our lives. A contemplative mind can help you open your mind to greater freedom and love. Tolle (2006) says that 98% of human thoughts are repetitive and meaningless. He believes that we are often unfree and says we need to have contact with our spiritual sources. We name the sources differently, based on the spiritual, religious or philosophical beliefs we belong to. These experiences can make us feel at home in the world, we are held by something bigger, and we have a mission in life. Maybe having a non-judgmental attitude and an open mind can help us be more loving in the sessions. Maybe it can help us be more friendly to the unfamiliar, being more open and curious.

Having a contemplative mind helps us listen to the body (Merleau-Ponty, 2002). The body can give us important knowledge about ourselves and our relationship with the world. By listening to the body, we become better therapists. Through it, we can live and work with what closes an open dialogue. Clients will easily sense if we are not open to their spiritual world (Holmberg, 2018; Holmberg et al., 2021). In systemic practice, we are not there only with our minds, but also with our hearts, body, feelings and creativity. We believe a relaxed and reflective relationship with our spirituality can make it easier for the clients to share their spiritual life.

Based on the development of the earth, we see that we need a new way of being in the world, which embodies the reality that life is sacred and valuable, and that we are connected. Contemplation can help us develop this awareness, an awareness that is necessary for shaping a more loving and sustainable world.

Closing Reflections

Moving back to the stories of the youths, we see that the young have a longing to be something for others. Perhaps it is then, when we stand in the suffering, that the spiritual emerges more clearly for us. Schnell (2011) says that research shows that generativity is established as the strongest predictor of meaningfulness. It means that you live in a way that affects the world or the lives of those who come after you. We know that loneliness is one of the great challenges of our time, so how can we as therapists work to ensure that people are connected more strongly and can experience that they mean something to others? Here, therapists can reflect more broadly helping clients to find ways within cultural life, religious contexts or other initiatives in society at large.

The young have many existential and spiritual reflections on life. They have a longing to also talk to professionals about this but feel that there is no room for this in the professional systems. As systemic therapists, we are aiming to embrace a holistic approach to life, where the spiritual part of humans may be included (Sheehan et al., 2007). We value an appreciative, dialogue-based practice where we are concerned with clients' perspectives and lives. We look for a pattern that connects, what gives meaning to humans' life. We say these perspectives also have to include the spiritual, religious and existential person. We need to show curiosity and openness to these topics as well. This is systemic work.

References

Andersen, H. (1997). *Conversation, language, and possibilities: A postmodern approach to therapy* (p. XIX, 308). Basic Books.

Andersen, T. (2011). *Reflekterande processer: samtal och samtal om samtalen [Reflective processes: conversations and conversations about conversations]* (5. uppl., p. 237). Studentlitteratur.

Bateson, G. (2000). *Steps to an ecology of mind* (p. XXXII, 533). University of Chicago Press.

Bateson, G., & Bateson, M. C. (1987). *Angels fear: Towards an epistemology of the sacred* (p. XII, 224). Macmillan.

Dallos, R., & Vetere, A. (2022). *Systemic therapy and attachment narratives: Applications in a range of clinical settings* (2nd ed.). Routledge.

Holmberg, Å. (2018). *Making room for spirituality? Family therapists' and clients' perceptions and experiences about spirituality in family therapy* (Vol. 9, p. XX, 285). VID Specialized University.

Holmberg, Å., Jensen, P., & Ulland, D. (2017). To make room or not to make room: Clients' narratives about exclusion and inclusion of spirituality in family therapy practice. *Australian and New Zealand Journal of Family Therapy, 38*(1), 15–26.

Holmberg, Å., Jensen, P., & Vetere, A. (2021). Spirituality–a forgotten dimension? Developing spiritual literacy in family therapy practice. *Journal of Family Therapy, 43*(1), 78–95.

https://cac.org/daily-meditations/

https://iep.utm.edu/goldrule/

Jensen, P. (2008). *The Narratives which connect…: A qualitative research approach to the Narratives which connect therapists' personal and private lives to their family therapy practices* (p. XI, 254). The University of East London.

Martinsen, K. (2005). Sårbarheten og omveiene: Løgstrup og sykepleien. In *Løgstrups mange ansigter [Vulnerability and detours: Løgstrup and nursing. Many faces of Løgstrup]* (pp. 255–269).

Merleau-Ponty, M. (2002). *Phenomenology of perception* (p. XXIV, 544). Routledge.

Miller, W. R., & Thoresen, C. E. (2003). Spirituality, religion, and health: An emerging research field. *American Psychologist, 58*(1), 24.

Rohr, R. (2014). *Eager to love: The alternative way of Francis of Assisi.* Franciscan Media.

Rosa, H. (2019). *Resonance: A sociology of our relationship to the world.* John Wiley & Sons.

Schibbye, A. L. L. (2009). *Relasjoner: Et dialektisk perspektiv på eksistensiell og psykodynamisk psykoterapi [Relationships: A dialectical perspective on existential and psychodynamic psychotherapy].* Universitetsforlaget.

Schnell, T. (2011). Individual differences in meaning-making: Considering the variety of sources of meaning, their density and diversity. *Personality and Individual Differences, 51*(5), 667–673. https://doi.org/10.1016/j.paid.2011.06.006

Seikkula, J. (2008). Inner and outer voices in the present moment of family and network therapy. *Journal of Family Therapy, 30,* 478–491.

Serander, E. (2018). När kroppen viser vägen. I: Stiwne, D. (red.) *Existens och psykisk hälsa- om hur liv och levnad förhåller sig till hälsa och ohälsa [Existence and mental health - how life and living relate to health and illness].* Studentlitteratur.

Sheehan, J., Flaskas, C., & McCarthy, I. (2007). *Hope and despair in narrative and family therapy: Adversity, forgiveness, and reconciliation* (p. XIII, 178). Routledge.

Swinton, J. (2001). *Spirituality and mental health care: Rediscovering a "forgotten" dimension* (p. 221). Jessica Kingsley Publishers.

Tolle, E. (2006). *New earth: Awakening to your life's purpose.* Penguin Life.

Tønder, E.S. & Karlsson, B.E. (2020). Resonans i relasjoner [Resonance in relations]. I: Buus, N., Askham, B., Berring, L. L., Hybholt, L., Stjernegaard, K., & Tønder, E. S. Psykiatrisk sygepleje (2. udgave.) (s.375–s.398). Munkgsaard.

Walsh, F. (2009). *Spiritual resources in family therapy* (2nd ed., p. XIX, 412). Guilford Press.

7

The Gift of Literary Fiction to Systemic Training and Practice

Anne Øfsti

My First Reading Experiences

In conjunction with my recent 60th birthday I received an envelope from my parents with black-and-white photographs from my childhood. In one of the photos I am sitting in the lower bunk together with my two younger siblings, all wearing flannel pyjamas. Next to the bunk bed mother is sitting in a stick chair, reading aloud. Perhaps it was the story of the ugly duckling by H.C. Andersen, or maybe we were listening to one of the wonderful tales of the mountain that opened up and tables being magically set. Open sesame, abracadabra and suddenly anything was possible. The book my mother was reading did not have many pictures in it, but I could see it all before me; two-headed trolls, princesses in four-poster beds and the tale of the fox's widow with her many suitors. The ritual was a gathering force; the sibling group was welded together in this

A. Øfsti (✉)
VID Specialized University, Oslo, Norway
e-mail: anne.ofsti@vid.no

peaceful hour before sleep. We received the message that the forces of Good conquer everything, and in the world of fairy tales anything is possible. When listening to these stories, a three-year-old imagines something different than a seven-year-old, and thus the shared reading experience created both a sense of belonging and development of different experiences, at the same time. Later, I experienced the freedom of reading for myself, what I wanted, when I wanted, and my little world expanded. It became possible to immerse myself in the lives of others, and curiosity about how lives can be lived in such different ways was awoken and stimulated. To me, the library became a wonderful oasis and a paradise. I would assert that reading fiction became more formative for who I am today, as a human being and as a therapist, than both nature and nurture. I am all those stories that I've read and heard. To me, this was especially significant, since I am adopted from a foreign country. I came to Norway in the early 1960s and had no stories about myself and my first years of life in Korea. Being a first-generation adoptee in an all-white Norway was demanding. There was a lack of stories about how you, as an adopted child, become a full-fledged member of a family in which everyone looks different from you, and where all the other kids are the biological offspring of your adoptive parents. Adult strangers would ask me: *Aren't you grateful for having come to Norway? Don't you miss your true mother?* These reactions are an expression of several things. first and foremost ignorance, and secondly a confirmation that one can never become "Norwegian enough", and being an adopted child is only the second best thing. Blood is thicker than water. The children of the orphanages are a genre of their own, with Annie, Oliver Twist and Anne of Green Gables. In different ways, their stories paint pictures of fate, betrayal, loneliness and a fragile sense of belonging. The stories of the children who received new families as an act of mercy offer different interpretations and repertoires for empathizing, while simultaneously creating a moral and existential space for action, for the adoptive families. And thus, *Anne of Green Gables* became my first reading pleasure through recognition. Anne's fear of being sent back to that orphanage, and her vital survival force, were crucial to me. And at the same time, the moral of the book was demanding; as an adoptee one must be charming, talented, and strive for amiability—a subtle message about adapting in order to avoid creating problems for the adoptive parents. But what touched me most deeply in the story of Anne of Green Gables was her wonderful imagination. In the midst of her cold and miserable reality she was able to conjure beauty and hope, making everything come alive and escaping into the magic of imagination and the power of daydreaming.

Longing for Home

In my years as a student I read psychology, philosophy and social anthropology; fields that, in different ways, provided insight into questions of what it means to be human, to belong. Texts with a focus on explaining, rather than experiencing. And do not get me wrong, I fell in love with theories, with existential philosophy, I read Freud with an ecstatic feeling of conquering insight. The theories became compasses to orient myself by, and I became a true believer in the scientific approach. After completing my degree as a social worker, I chose to study family therapy. I occasionally get asked why I wanted to become a family therapist, and the answer is both many-faceted and perhaps very simple. I believe I have been suffering from homesickness all my life, that a part of me is related to the child in *The Little Match Girl* of Hans Christian Anderson, who stands out in the dark night looking through the window at the family that is gathered around the table, with lit candles and food on the table. My homesickness is of the sentimental, melancholic sort. I still enjoy wandering the streets after dark, looking into the bright rooms, fantasizing about the lives in there, who they are, how they are doing, what they are doing right now. Still, literature has, to me, been the most generous window into the lives of others, and it has been liberating to read stories devoid of narrow categories, such as dysfunctional interactions or disoriented attachment. The window of literature shows how complex we humans are, how fragilely we live, in different circumstances, and how strongly we fight and love. My own family tried hard to be a completely normal family, but did not quite make it. My family's struggles gave me plenty of experiential competence: I learned how painful it can be when conflicts arise in what should be one's safe space, and the joy that can be found in glimpses of reconciliation and moving forward in fragile relationships. In addition to curiosity and a longing for stories about my own and others' lives, I felt the desire to become a therapist as a *calling*, in the same way that priests and politicians might feel called upon. It may sound ostentatious, but to me this is about a deep and sincere wish to use language as a mean to forming porous attachments, heal broken connections and make people function together in the imperfect group of which they are part.

And, inspired by the wish to become a family therapist, I travelled to Kirkenes, at the northern tip of Norway, with northern lights, polar nights and the midnight sun. To a former mining village, where most families were alike, heterosexual couples with two to three children. A family resembling my own, in many ways, and also families in novels I had read. Stored deeply within my soul was the reading about happy families, as in *Little House on the Prairie*, and other post-war novels, where the nuclear family is presented as the only true way of belonging. Being a therapist in the early nineteen nineties was nice, it felt meaningful, I helped the families stick together in spite of quarrels, infidelity and disagreements over how much sex one should expect in a marriage. I settled on the belief that the meaning of being human is to create a family, make it into a nest, a shelter, against the cold and dark.

What Does It Mean to Live Separately and Together?

Ten years later I started to work as a therapist near Oslo, with its continental climate and big city pulse. Something had happened to the expectations to cohabitation, the script of family life had changed, it was not characterized by quite the same harmony and unity as before. In those days I was reading coming-of-age novels that confronted the image of the idyllic nuclear family. The metaphor about the family as a safe haven was now morphed into an unsafe, claustrophobic arena. In Norway, authors like Hanne Ørstavik and Trude Marstein have been especially prominent in depicting tragic relationships between children and their parents. In Ørstavik's *Tiden det tar* (*The Time It Takes*), Ørstavik (2000) the daughter Signe confronts her parents on the subject of celebrating Christmas:

Why do you have to pressure me, I said. Mom sighed.

–

I don't understand why you must pressure me into
participating in your Christmas, I said. I began to cry. […]

–

We were so afraid,
and we were all alone. Mom looked at me as if I were telling a lie.
Dad got up from the sofa, he walked round the table and came toward me.

–

But Signe, he said and stood beside
Mom in front of me, he bent down and spoke with a soft voice.

–

Were you afraid? What was
it you were afraid of? He cocked his head, the little smile about his lips, his
eyes were hard
and small […] Everything I had been thinking disappeared, I heard a loud,
high-pitched note, as if a strong wind was blowing […]

–

If you believe, Signe, [Mom] began, she spoke slowly.

–

If you believe that this is the whole story,
you are mistaken. […]

–

You mustn't believe that you possess the truth. […] There was nothing to
say, I had said
everything, and it was as if I had said nothing. (pp. 44–45, translated from
Norwegian)

And at the same time, I was devouring feminist authors who fought
their way out of destructive partnerships, to be replaced by an (often rau-
cous) freedom. These descriptions of conflict resolution made a deep
impression on me. After reading authors like Marilyn French, I would lie

awake, shaken, agitated and tender. The literary uprising against the nuclear family and the conventional romantic couple was also reflected in the therapy room. Couples were no longer primarily fighting over house chores, economy and child-rearing. Now, the very existence and justification of the relationship itself was exposed to doubt. The questions were existentially and ethically formulated, and thus the field of couples therapy began turning towards philosophy and poetry, in addition to being an area for normative theories and psychological models of attachment. Can infidelity be forgiven? Are we supposed to live in a loveless relationship, out of consideration for the children? Can we continue in a sexless relationship?

And the questions I asked myself were: Which sources of knowledge are available and, even more importantly, most suitable for the exploration of the character of these issues?

Late modernity is characterized by changes in the forms of intimacy; we move from solid, predictable structures to fluid relationships (Beck & Beck-Gernsheim, 1995), as a consequence of several processes of liberation and revolutionary changes in society, economic growth, feminism, individualization, globalization, democratization and secularization. Or, more simply put, individuals gain more freedom to choose their way of life, the nuclear family becomes more prone to disintegration and thus therapeutic practices change. And with changed practices one needs new stories about how to live with new forms of intimacy. One of the most important characteristics of the new forms of intimacy is the ideal of mental intimacy, communication and self-realization. From a more traditional perspective on gender roles to what is called pure relationships (Giddens, 1992), where the inherent value of the relationship is considered most important, and which is not driven by duty, tradition or economic companionship. In the Norwegian contemporary literature, these questions that couples struggle with are reflected. One example is the novel *Elin og Hans* (Marstein, 2002), in which Hans asks himself after the breakup:

> Why didn't we take better care of what we had together?
> Why did we allow what we had together to slowly die out? (Marstein, 2002) translated from Norwegian)

In my doctoral thesis *Some Call It Love* (Øfsti, 2008), I investigated what kind of knowledge family therapists need and utilize when faced with existential and ethical issues. There was one observation in particular that had a formative effect on my scientific work, and it came about through an encounter with a couple in their fifties who expressed doubt about the continuation of their relationship. They had everything they could wish for, and yet they were unsure of whether they wanted to continue as a couple. The doubt affected them both, and they took turns expressing it. I explored stories from their childhoods, intimacy, emotionality, patterns of attachment and their history of couples therapy in order to gauge whether their relationship was strong enough to continue. The evening before one of my last sessions with them I had been to the cinema and watched a movie about forbidden love and the fiery passion that follows such a narrative, and it felt like a mental catharsis and awakening to me. The next day, when faced with the couple, it was as though every nerve of my body wished to convey to them that the relationship they had was too indifferent and dull. I wanted to awaken their passion and tell them that true love exists. Of course I never said any of this, but I am sure that some of the fallout from my own awakening leaked into the conversation. The discovery became significant because I understood that on the subject of love, the most vital sources of knowledge come from fiction, art and lived life. Knowledge of love is found in representations of what we, culturally, historically and contextually, present it as.

Literary Fiction: A Tuning Fork for Sensitivity

Paradoxically, after having completed my doctoral I arrived at the acknowledgement that the academic language was too categorical. It made me feel unfree, and as though removed from my practice as a therapist. In 2014 I published the novel *Si at vi har hele dagen* (*If We Only Had All Day*) (Øfsti, 2014) through Gyldendal publishing house. This novel explored my own story of memories, sorrow and belonging from my experience of being adopted. During the writing process I discovered the ability of language to touch and disturb all the way down to the microlevel. I learned to make the language seem tender, to create powerful life. Our imagination is a source that needs nourishment. I will never forget the discovery I made during a meeting with a couple who taught me the effect of language at the micro-level. A sorrowful encounter. The woman was ill with cancer and nine months pregnant and was being kept alive long enough for the child to be born. The couple had great difficulties talking to one another—while also expressing the need to do precisely this—without being overwhelmed by emotion or just falling silent. I was invited to come by the oncology nurse. Normally, we therapists ask our clients: *What would you like to talk about?* In this grave situation I felt that such a question would be too cliche. I asked:

> What *must* you talk about?
> We m*ust* talk about names, he replied.

And thus the conversation got started, there was some cautious laughter—and I asked him another question:

> What are you going to do now, for the next hour?
> I'm going shopping for some baby clothes, he said.
> What kind of clothes? I asked.
> A pair of rompers, she whispered.
> Yes, he said, and turned to me. And afterwards we will take pictures so the child can see Mom with the rompers.

Here, the minor words are effective at keeping the present moment alive. *Must* and *will* are words that take hold of the couple, and bring them into an impossible future, if only for a little bit. This is the language awareness that comes from that poetry, that literary source, that which goes into the particulars, into the relationship, into their very special situation and yet connects it with a collective loneliness, the great death, the little death, the almost wordless.

The Journal, the Novel and Their Different Voices

In the professional fields, there is disagreement over the theories, research and evidence-based knowledge and therapy models. Knowing and understanding that there is power and economics involved in any field of knowledge, is necessary. In the field of family therapy, new manual-based and evidence-based models come along and are implemented in different settings, including child protective services, family protection, education and mental healthcare, by the power elite. Professional knowledge has become profit-based and market-oriented. The different evidence-based texts gain their status as evident and eminent over literature and art. This may not be problematic in and of itself, but a closer look at this production of text reveals that the underlying motivation is about generalization and effectivization. We need academic knowledge in order to motivate our activity, and we need scientific texts that can espouse knowledge that is valid for more than the singular. But we also need, as a vaccine against the generalization, literary fiction, poetry, autoethnographic texts and, for that matter, dance and movement without words. In Liz Burns' (2009) book *Literature and Therapy*, she explores and grapples with similar themes to those that I raise.

Literary fiction has expanded to become something we read in our spare time, individually and as a private matter. As part of our family therapeutic study programme, we once invited the now deceased author Beate Grimsrud. At the end of the day, she asked me: *What should we do to get the students to read novels?* In 2010 Grimsrud published the novel *En dåre fri (A Free Fool)* (Grimsrud, 2010). The main character, Eli, initially presents herself as follows:

> "I'm Eli. It means God in Hebrew. It's both a boy's name and a girl's name."
> Eli conducts inner conversations with several voices, such as Espen, Emil, Erik, Prince Eugen. Eli is the first-person voice.

Eli conducts inner conversations with several voices, such as Espen, Emil, Erik and Prince Eugen. Eli is the first-person narrator. She suffers from serious mental anguish and yet she is a creative writer, she makes movies, books and plays. Her voice is appealing and interesting, we are pulled into her universe, and simultaneously get to hear how she at times is attacked by intrusive thoughts and ideas, which lead her to self-harm and different attempts to escape the pain. In the novel a different voice emerges: *From the journal.*

Pt. got agitated last night. Threw glasses in the dining hall, said she would cut herself. She said she would hurt herself and hit her head against the wall. An employee sat with her for a long time, but a straitjacket was eventually necessary.

In this text Eli's name is no longer Eli, but "pt.", and the subject disappears in the last sentence, which ends in a pronouncement:

> An employee sat with her for a long time, but a straitjacket was eventually necessary.

And in the next passage the objectification from the journal is reinforced:

> Pt. has clearly hallucinatory experiences. Pt. is motorically agitated during the conversation, shaking her legs, hitting her head against the wall, suddenly laughing etc.

Eli's voice comes as a follow-up in the text:

> I want to go home. I want to get out of Erik. Out into the fresh air and the coming heat. The summer that no longer reaches into the ward. I want to go home to Eli who decides.

Sørbø (2013) points to Foucault—who, in *Madness and Civilization*, explores the point in history where insanity and normality were not separated. Foucault writes:

> The constitution of madness as a mental illness, at the end of the eighteenth century, affords the evidence of a broken dialogue, posits the separation as already effected, and thrusts into oblivion all those stammered, imperfect words without fixed syntax in which the exchange between madness and reason was made. The language of psychiatry, which is a monologue of reason *about* madness, has been established only on the basis of such a silence. I have not tried to write the history of that language, but rather the archaeology of that silence. (Foucault, 1988, p. 10)

Sæbønes points to the existence of a third party, who falls in neither with the monologue of sense nor with the illness of silence: this is literary fiction. In Grimsrud's novel neither delusions nor compulsions are denied, but the dividing line between madness and normalcy is not an absolute, objective one.

I problematize the textual hierarchy and point to the necessity of writing, allowing for and highlighting alternative texts when it comes to therapy, treatment, hope and change. If we get too many texts of the sort that generalize human experience, that make numerical arguments, trim away meaning and sweep away wonder and hope in the field of therapy, damages may result. We may start to imagine that we know more than we can know, and forget that there exists a diversity of lived life, that life itself doesn't always add up, even when one lives by the book.

We need texts to be written, therapeutic, or literary for that matter, which speak to the exceptional case, to the human experience—to the one who lives, or that which is lived, marginally on the fringe. We need therapeutic texts that don't pretend to represent the general, what we think we can know with certainty (Øfsti, 2013, translated from Norwegian).

Bringing Literature Groups into the Study of Family Therapy

In the training study programme *Master of Family Therapy and Systemic Practice* we have agreed that it is important to bring literary fiction into the programme. The attitude towards literature as being important, but not important enough, reflects a general trend in our society. We have become a non-literary culture, writes Marstein (2002) and quotes Hans Magnus Enzensberger who explains the down-prioritization of literature in society as a consequence of its loss of utility: it does not provide social status, nor is it able to serve anyone's (capitalist) interests, and it has no real place in the education programmes of the state. And, according to Enzensberger, we now have a new kind of illiteracy: High-ranking leader figures in politics and business who can produce case documents, but have no visions and thoughts of their own about how the world should be. When I read this, I thought it could be relevant to the field of therapy as well, how knowledge and science are produced mainly from a profit-based perspective, and less so based on values and free thought about what therapy can and should be. Students go through the training study programme, and we talk about portfolio and points, often detached from cultural history, literature and tradition. And yet, without being able to document this, I seem to sense a warm literary wind blowing into our society, our institutions and academic circles; perhaps as a counterbalance to the authoritarian texts, perhaps as part of a yearning towards gathering around the "campfire". This led us to establish a new subject in our training study programme: Literature groups inspired by Shared Reading.

Shared Reading is a literature-based practice developed by The Reader, an organization based in Liverpool, where small groups gather to read literature together and share personal experiences connected to this literature. The participants become engaged in a dialogue whose foremost characteristic is that it plays out around literature as a live presence and emotional centre (as opposed to merely objects of analysis). Shared Reading is applied in different institutional contexts such as public libraries, hospitals, psychiatric wards, prisons and senior centres and in educational contexts.

Report from One of the Literature Groups

This early morning it had been snowing all night, and the scenery outside looked like an old-fashioned Christmas card. And I was happy for that little moment of nostalgia, of belonging, and the air of expectation. I have always had an ambivalent relationship with the Christmas holiday, with its high expectations of joy, and a little too many experiences of collapse even before dinner on Christmas Eve. And yet, I have a recurring wish for the glimpses of the Christmas joy of my childhood to reappear and be real as well.

In the classroom, the air was rich with the scent of wet wool, mandarins and freshly brewed coffee. We sat down in a circle with no tables. I had made an arrangement with student R in advance, she was to read aloud: the short story *Julaften* ("Christmas Eve") by Vigdis Hjorth (Hjorth, 2021).

The story revolves around a mother who is about to celebrate Christmas with her adult children. There is an air of excitement and expectation about the text: Will someone get too drunk? The mother finds her children surveilling her, paying attention to her alcohol consumption. She must not drink, and she drinks. R reads:

> A nervousness accompanies the children's expectations, which increases the thirst. Preferably I would have been drinking since morning. But that wouldn't work. I mustn't get drunk. If I get drunk, it will all be ruined, it will be awful, all the days they're staying here, arguing, crying, impossible. I mustn't get drunk. There's nothing more thirst-inducing than that. I won't make it without drinking, but I mustn't get drunk. (Hjorth, 2021, translated from Norwegian)

As R keeps reading about the main character—this mother, who constantly fights an inner fight against the bottle, who makes excuses to go down to the basement where she has hidden some cans of apple cider—I look around. Most of the students are looking down, looking out the window, none meet my gaze, some are writing by themselves, but it is an active, listening silence, as silent as snow falling upon snow.

> The youngest daughter calls and says she's on her way. I'm sure she won't be drinking. She has a strained relationship with alcohol. She saves her drinking for parties with friends. When she's with us, her family, she doesn't drink. She's damaged […] My son asks if she would like a beer. My ears perk up, I hope she'll say yes, that she'll drink many beers and a lot of wine and forget about me, so I can get drunk. I wish everyone would get drunk and lose themselves in gifts and forget about me. She shakes her head, she doesn't want any beer, it's the damage. (Hjorth, 2021, translated from Norwegian)

After this paragraph we take a break from reading aloud and the conversation begins. I, as the group leader, ask a few introductory questions about where we are in the story, who is present and what the text is about. What is at stake for the main character and how the inner monologue can be interpreted? The conversation is open and immediate when it comes to the more "factual" parts of the text. The conversation also flows relatively easily when it comes to how the inner dialogue can be understood. Several of the students say they feel touched by the inner struggle of the main character, that they can almost understand her desperation for drinking, and that they feel the struggle as a sense of unease in the body. Other students find it hard to understand that she is not more concerned with her children, and feel resentment. They, too, say that they feel the unease in their bodies. When we come to the question of message, open and subtle, all go quiet before the first voices pipe up to say that they perceive the subtle message to be ambiguous. Some opine that the reader is meant to feel how strong the thirst is—and that the message is to trigger empathy with such a thirst and such a love of intoxication. Others thought that the implicit message had to do with understanding how taxing it is to the adult children to have to watch how their mother handles her own alcohol abuse. We also dwelt upon the word *damage*, and how we can understand the term relationally. Does the damage consist in mistrust, betrayal, all the bad memories, and is it irreparable? At this point it was clear that strong emotions had been set in motion, and most of the students took the perspective of the adult children, but some also wanted to explore how the mother does seem to manage herself—and how she is open and honest about her struggle, which is valuable in itself. One of the students said there was something liberating about the mother's openness, that there are too many hypocrites when it comes to alcohol use. This in turn brought up the subject of intoxication as generosity, rather than the "boring" teetotaller aunt who sours whole parties with her strict way of life.

The student R reads on, and the last sentences of the short story are as follows:

> I go down to my room and shut the door. Sit down on the bed, open the nice, expensive bottle as a reward. Find the nicest glass, pour, drink greedily. I didn't get drunk, now I can get drunk. Light a fire in the fireplace, put on clean pajamas, sit down on the bed, they won't come, I've gone to bed, I've called it a night, they won't know what I'm doing. It's gone well, now I can drink. The bed is freshly made, I drink and watch the fire and have more wine in the locker. It's done, it's over with, I'm by myself, finally, happily. (Hjorth, 2021, translated from Norwegian)

After R had finished reading, it got quiet. She looked up at the rest of us, I met her gaze, she seemed moved, happy to have read aloud, to have had us listen. I looked up and around the circle, some were blushing, one of the students avoided my gaze and seemed very uncomfortable. What now, I asked. The subjects from earlier were picked up again. It was as though the group split in two: those who empathized with the mother and those who were morally outraged. Several brought up experiences from their work, and some identified with the adult children. The atmosphere was emotional and charged, and in this sense I believe the short story brings up certain qualities that a therapist needs: empathy with what seems incomprehensible, identification with one's own discomfort, insight into the fragile dilemmas around boundaries and boundary crossing, and contact with themes that show the vulnerability of the parent-child relationship, tied to expectation and betrayal. After talking about how the text touched us, we did a writing exercise. *Write a letter or poem for one of the characters in the short story, where you assume the role of a witness, where you share of yourself, and where you try to avoid being interpretive or an observer.*

Letters were written both for the mother and for the children. One of the students, who had been the most appalled by the mother's selfishness, wrote a letter where she tried to be empathetic. The letter went as follows: *Dear mother, I do not understand you, I can't understand that your thirst is your main focus on Christmas Eve, and yet it's as though I sense your joy, that you're finally free, when you are alone and can drink. I don't wish to judge you, because I believe you were struggling with your own demons throughout the night, and that you managed to be considerate enough of your children that you didn't get drunk, but managed to wait.*

The greatest value in the literature groups, as I see it, is that the students read life themes *with* the characters in the stories, and not *about*. It becomes relational, encounters between fictional people, and not objective clients. Something happens in this encounter, points of contact arise, in little leaks between the characters and the lives of the students. Hopefully this can make the students more wondering, less cocksure, more participating in everything that isn't documented in forms, but which, at the end of the day, revolves around how aesthetics and ethics make us more human. I believe that seeking an ancient ritual creates forms of belonging and growth, which does something to a learning atmosphere. And I like to think about the slowness in the time it takes to read aloud, as a contemplation in an otherwise performance-oriented culture that expects efficiency. I hope and believe that this slowness can whisper forth the third voice, which in this case, where the mother in the short story is both a caring mother (she doesn't want to let her children down, she knows how important it is to them that she doesn't get drunk) and yet at her happiest when she is alone and free to drink. A kind of homesickness, that too.

References

Beck, U., & Beck-Gernsheim, E. (1995). *The normal chaos of love*. Polity Press.

Burns, L. (2009). *Literature and therapy. A systemic view*. Routledge.

Foucault, M. (1988). *Madness and civilization: A history of insanity in the age of reason*. Vintage Books.

Giddens, A. (1992). *The transformation of intimacy: Sexuality, love and eroticism in modern societies*. Polity Press.

Grimsrud, B. (2010). *En dåre fri* [A free fool]. Cappelen Damm.

Hjorth, V. (2021). *Julaften* [Christmas Eve]. Samlaget.

Marstein, T. (2002). *Elin og Hans* [Elin og Hans]. Oktober forlag.

Øfsti, A. (2014). *Si at vi har hele dagen* [If we only had the all day]. Gyldendal.

Øfsti, A. K. S. (2008). *Some call it love. Exploring Norwegian systemic couple therapists discourses of love, intimacy and sexuality 2008*. University of East London.

Øfsti, A. K. S. (2013) Å lese etter teksten - Om teksters betydning for terapeutisk praksis, om å være leser og skriver av tekster om terapi, trøst og forandring [To be a reader and writer in therapeutic practice – For comfort and change]. *Fokus på familien*, (1), 5–18.

Ørstavik, H. (2000). *Tiden det tar*. Oktober forlag.

Sørbø, J. I. (2013). *Til trøyst* [To comfort]. Samlaget.

8

Till Life Do Us Apart: An Exploration of Crumbs on the Floor and Existential Themes in Couples Therapy

Sigurd Riste Andersen
and Thomas Bernhard Thiis-Evensen

Introduction

In couples therapy, as in life itself, it is impossible to avoid certain fundamental challenges, doubts, dilemmas and questions. These might involve themes like identity, meaning, sickness and death, freedom, responsibility, choice, remorse, guilt, shame, loneliness, relations and attachment (Yalom, 1980). As a therapist, we assume you already meet and work with such themes and relate to and address such challenges in various ways in meeting with couples. We understand these themes to be existential and, in this chapter, we will show how we might explore such phenomena in an existential way. We will also explore some of the ways in

S. R. Andersen (✉)
VID Specialized University, Oslo, Norway
e-mail: Sigurd.andersen@vid.no

T. B. Thiis-Evensen
Board of Education, Norwegian Society of Philosophical Practice (NSFP),
Oslo, Norway

T. Grover et al. (eds.), *New Horizons in Systemic Practice with Adults*, Palgrave Texts in Counselling and Psychotherapy, https://doi.org/10.1007/978-3-031-30526-9_8

which we respond to the following questions as they emerge in our work. In our own experience with meeting couples, many of the topics brought up in therapy have an implicit grounding in existential themes. So, how can we help couples make the implicit explicit, to better work towards their goals of therapy and a shared horizon?

This chapter combines relational, systemic theory with existential perspectives. It will describe how existential themes are an essential and natural part of systemic work with couples. We also argue that existential themes should be given a bigger role in relational, systemic work and should be a part of further development in the field of family therapy. This chapter will to a lesser degree explain *what* existential therapy might be said to be, as this is covered well in other books (van Deurzen & Arnold-Baker, 2018). The goal is rather to show what the exploration of existential experiences might be said to *do* with couples, what they might *mean* and *how* exploration of fundamental questions might benefit a couple's relationship.

After a short introduction, we will describe our work with a couple to show relevant theory in practice. We will bring forward an existential theme from the therapy to show how we can address such topics in therapy. We hope to inspire you as a practitioner to reflect on how you recognize existential themes and how you might address them. We hope you will enjoy the chapter.

Our Own Life Experiences

As writers we acknowledge the dialogue between this text and our own life experiences. I, Sigurd, have gone through different life challenges, encountered death and break-ups and am dealing with various questions of meaning. This has made me reflect on my own life, but also to be more curious about how couples I meet in therapy relate to the fundamental themes in their life, and what they expect from their partner. I, Thomas Bernhard, have experienced the loss of a family member when young, and have experienced how traumatic life events influence a family. Finding ways to practise dialogue on existential themes as a way of experiencing recovery and empowerment has been a leitmotif.

Cultural Context and Background

In an individualistic time and culture, we are fed information and answers on how to cope with everyday life or deal with close relations: how to be a good parent, partner, throwing away unnecessary items or lowering our stress levels. Through media and input our culture makes us receivers of information, rather than participants in self-involved, phenomenological exploration of them (Skjervheim, 1996). In therapy we might experience that clients are asking for tools or placing the therapist in an expert position. Different traditions, models and manuals are fighting over telling us they have the answers, but have we forgotten what the questions are, and what it takes to answer them?

Still, existential themes seem to be increasingly relevant in our culture (Binder, 2020). Parallel to the constant machinations of the answering-bots of self-help culture, we have met many families, couples and individuals during and after the Covid-19 pandemic that have experienced a need to ask more fundamental questions. Many have experienced rapid changes no one saw coming, isolation from friends and family, and have gone through processes of cherishing other sources of meaning in life, differently from before. Many have put stronger value on the quality of certain relations, and what may be important in an involved and self-reflexive, uncertain life. We are living in a time of environmental crisis, big cultural differences and a war in Europe for the first time since World War II. Parallel with an individualistic culture and materialistic focus it seems that existential themes are coming more to the fore (Thorsted & Hansen, 2022). As Åse Homberg writes in a different chapter in this book, many people are experiencing a need for exploring their own spirituality. Perhaps we are currently on our way towards leaving some of the materialistic/mechanistic answers to life's questions behind and going back to explore new answers in the complexity of our relations and a bigger, relational and existential whole?

The Couple

We will use the following example from the therapy room to show how various existential themes might emerge in a session. We will further show how we might explore the themes together with the couple, possibly contributing to understanding and a strengthening of the bond between the two. The example is anonymous and is loosely based on reality.

Melody and Margot are two women that have been in a relationship for 3 years. Melody is 33 and Margot is 42 years of age. Margot has an 8-year-old son from an earlier relationship. They contact a private therapist and describe that they are happy with their relationship in many ways, but recently have experienced more arguing and conflicts that escalate into several days of disconnection. They want help communicating better and avoiding conflicts that could last for days. The two describe their differences and agree on Melody being the more outgoing and socially oriented of the two, while Margot tends to prefer spending time at home with her son or watching a film together with Melody. The couple is currently living in a bigger city where Melody enjoys the opportunities of going to clubs and meeting up with friends.

They are describing what they see as their problems and what they are fighting about. Margot describes that they are in a slightly different situation in life. Margot has a child, but Melody does not need to take the same kind of consideration and responsibility for others. Margot feels somewhat lonely in her situation and refers to talks from the beginning of their relationship where they discussed sharing the responsibility for her son. In addition, Margot would consider having another child, both for her son to have a sibling, but also to share this experience with Melody.

Melody on the other hand is reluctant to have children and is hesitant to how a child would limit her way of living and social life. The two describe that the level of frustration is high when they argue and that they fight and get annoyed with each other for small things like washing the dishes. Melody describes that Margot's son is making a lot of mess and that the family life they represent is not very appealing.

Constant crumbs on the floor and a negative atmosphere annoys Melody and leads to her spending more time out of the house with friends than earlier. Margot expresses concern in spending less time together and is afraid this might be harmful to their relationship in the long run. They both describe a feeling of not being a good version of themselves and do not really understand what is going on. How did crumbs and the distribution of housework become so important? And how can they deal with the more fundamental questions in life, like having a child together or not. They ask the therapist for help in understanding how they can deal with their issues and bring them closer together.

How to Explore Existential Themes

Theoretical Introduction

As biologist Gregory Bateson describes systems theory and cybernetics, it is not possible to separate ourselves from others, not in the world, and not in therapy. We are part of an ecology of nature and are a part of a bigger, relational whole. We are self-reflexively creating meaning in context and are hence always dealing with questions of existence in relation to ourselves, something and/or someone. Whereas earlier psychotherapeutic practice, like psychoanalysis, saw the therapist as an objective observer of the system, the development of systemic therapy saw the therapist increasingly as *part* of the system. In our view, therapists are always in dialogue, both with the situation, our clients, but also with ourselves. In existential therapy we are confronted with our own fundamental concerns and anxiety in meeting with clients, because we are a part of a common journey.

Existential phenomena are factual, relational, deeply personal and holistic, they apply to all of us, and there are no clear-cut answers to the task they present us with. We are all experts in our own lives, and we "become who we are" (Nietzsche, 2001) through our attitude towards, our relating to and handling of existential themes. How do we describe what happens between two people, and a person and their world? Existential phenomenology is the attempt to meet and describe the world as it appears, as we concretely and specifically, bodily and existentially experience it. It is a way of practising knowledge seeking in situations, the world and being, that is open, wondering and explorative (Thorsted & Hansen, 2022).

One operative definition of the existential is that it: "concerns the way life and the conditions of life are experienced, given meaning to and managed by the individual" (Norwegian Directorate of Health, 2016).

In a workshop by Thomas Bernhard with a group of psychologists in a hospital in Norway in 2019, the group wanted to explore and find a feasible answer to the question "What is existential practice?" By working out the following common traits/factors based on an exemplary case of being therapeutic in an existential crisis, the group put their combined experience to use and found that *existential practice is:*

- *Being here, present, together*
- *Meeting one's own anxiety*
- *Enduring the wordless*
- *Seeking support in what enables you to be here for the other*
- *Having the courage to be present in what is as it is, despite resistance*
- *Contributing to the others ability to stand upright in their "mineness"*

These factors may clarify what we all always already do when trying to help someone near to us in a crisis. We are familiar with our way of doing this, as we have done it many times.

At the same time, it might explain why it is difficult working with existential health in a *professional* way. It is easy to understand the temptation to administer standard solutions or to narrow the scope to focus on better communication techniques. Communication is validated not only by the "how", but also by the "what"—what it lets emerge in a common horizon of interpretation. If existential practice demands our *authentic* presence, manifests *our own anxiety*, takes away our *language*, makes us seek our *personal strongholds* to overcome our *resistance against that which is as it is*, all for the sake of our patient's *ability to "own" their situation*, it is a wicked challenge, and one to be reckoned with.

Our own life might resonate through bodily sensations in confronting our own existential questions, and we are constantly punctuating, setting meaning to and making choices in various parts of a conversation. What are we avoiding in a session? We argue that many therapists, us included, subconsciously avoid certain questions or themes, simply because they awake discomfort or anxiety in us. But this discomfort or anxiety might on the other hand be a gift in the therapy room. If the disturbing feeling we get from our own existential concerns—our own fear of loneliness, death, meaninglessness, or freedom—how do we put it to good use? Maybe we are faced with the dilemma of what to ask next and feel the discomfort of all the choices we have to make. Or maybe we fear that our next question or intervention might sound simplistic to the other and give us a fear of rejection which might link to our own fear of loneliness and solitude? As therapists we could shift focus away from our own ideals of being "the good therapist", thus shielding ourselves from actually relating, to being more present with the clients as who we are, where they are, in a common exploration of important themes without clear-cut predefined answers.

Relating to Melody and Margot

As therapists we must dare to venture into the unknown and deal with the uncertain, self-involving and discomforting to help others in being open to their own experiences, being present, and to create new meaning. When Melody and Margot are describing their situation to us, we might feel resonance with our own life. Maybe we have recognized the feeling of being lonely, not getting what we expect from our partner or have been in situations where big decisions make us uncertain and overwhelmed.

For couples in therapy, personal insight and an understanding of various meaning dimensions might be of great value, both for oneself and a partner. Meaning is a premise for communication (Binder, 2020) and meaning systems are the foundation of self-reflections, choices, values and goals. Through language we create ways to understand and see the world and when we are born into the world we are born into stories of right and wrong and how the world can and should be understood. If we are present in an open and meaning-oriented way, our bodily sensations might tell us when these stories are on the verge of collapsing, and when something important is manifesting itself that we could explore further (Solvoll & Lindseth, 2016).

As described through second order cybernetics, the therapist is always a part of the system and what is going on in the therapy room. With the case of Melody and Margot, a comment like "when I listen to you, I feel my body getting more tense and I'm wondering if that is because I sense an existential concern that emerges when you feel disconnected in your fights". This might sound personal and private to share, but on the other hand it might contribute to the therapist being a role model for opening up on existential themes by addressing their own feelings or discomfort. This might create openness in the session and create new possibilities, intimacy and talks for the couple we are seeing. We then turn avoidance into a validation of resistance and a quality for the therapy. Through sharing our thoughts on the atmosphere, mood or themes of a session, the therapist could introduce a broader picture and create a space for exploration rather than striving to reach certain prefixed goals in the therapeutic process.

Exploring with Melody and Margot: Step by Step

The following exploration is loosely based on the method of Socratic dialogue (Hansen, 2015; Nelson, 1922). The method is a structured whole, here shortened to include what in our view is the most relevant for our context. Socratic dialogue is a phenomenological, narrative, hermeneutic and dialogical approach where the therapist has a not-knowing-position, and everyone's personal experiences and perspectives are equally valid. We thus form "a community of inquiry" (Garrison, 2015). This is a common search for insight into the phenomena the couple chooses to work with. What *is it*, what *does* it do to them, and *how* might they move forward?

As an invitation to an existential exploration for Melody and Margot, we could ask:

From what you have said, I understand that you are happy with your relationship in many ways, but experience some challenges lately and your goal is to communicate better, avoid conflicts, solve issues, reverse dissolving tendencies and be closer. Is that correct? When I hear you describing your situation, goals and your wonderment over what really stops you from reaching them, could I invite you to an exploration of these themes to see what possible answers we could work out to move towards your goal?

Through our conversations to now, I have become aware of some recurring existential questions and themes I would like to run by you, to check if we are on the same page, and if you think it could be useful to examine one or more of these themes in depth. Is that ok with you?

As Melody and Margot are happy to continue the conversation about this we might ask: We could explore your experience of some tasks life confronts us with, and questions that are both grounding in our lives, deeply personal, common to all although in a personal way, and without clear-cut answers. We often live as though we have the answers to these questions, but when we look closer or fight over them, we obviously do not, or at least we do not seem to have the same ones. By exploring together, we might be able to work on what you brought with you today and what you care about. If we are to explore a theme, we need to ask authentic questions (Hansen, 2008). Asking an authentic question means acknowledging the fact that you really do not know the answer, but that you want to, and are willing to work for it. Asking a question together in a community of inquiry (Garrison, 2015) od, 2015) means inviting the other to explore with you, laying bare their conception of their world, their identity and horizon of meaning as their gift to a common quest. Are you willing to do that?

Step 1: Creating a Community of Wonder and Finding an Existential Theme

We start the exploration with Margot and Melody by establishing curiosity and finding an existential theme together:

Humans are normally deeply involved in caring for ourselves, our important others, and our world. The way we do this is often grounded in our conception of the world, ourselves in relation to others, and what we think is important and meaningful. When experiencing something we really like, our "model of the good life" might be manifested in some way that could make us utter "ah, it is good to be, good to be me with my people, and things just make sense!". Do you know the feeling? On the other hand when things happen that threaten or shatter this "model of the good life", we might find it hard to properly care for our world, ourself and what's important to us, and we feel more lonely, anxious, that things are meaningless, and get overly sensitive and aggressive about things. Is this recognizable?

If someone asked you: Why do you want this relationship to work, and you wanted to give a really thorough answer, how would you do it, and what would you say, knowing you would witness your assumptions about your world, your relationship to yourself and others, and your horizon of meaning/value? Is there any particular theme that you think would be useful to examine experiences of together, to get you towards where you want, to get you closer to each other going forward?

Melody and Margot might suggest different themes and we might talk a bit about the different options in order to find the most useful one:

So you both get interested in the theme of "profound joy", I think that is a marvellous idea! One can focus on many things making one unhappy and learn a lot about the lack of good and important things, but not getting any closer to a common understanding of what joy is actually all about, for you. You said earlier you were "happy together in many ways", and exploring what really makes you happy might clarify what your individual "model of the good life" is, and what your common model going forward could be, and how to strengthen it.

Step 2: Find Events of Positive Manifestation of Phenomena and Choose One

We have all experienced joy, and "know" what joy is, but let's find some examples that could help us understand more of what happiness and joy is, does to us, and might mean!

Could both of you find three events where you personally experienced profound joy or happiness? A concrete situation where it was good to be, good to be you, and things had meaning? What happened? It is helpful if the event is simple, happened in a short timespan, is ok to share and lay out for common inquiry, and does not have to have a clear bearing on what might be difficult right now (then it becomes counselling, and not exploration), and it might be useful if it happened a long time ago, because if you still remember it, it might be important.

So to find out more about what joy is, could each of you share two or three short descriptions of situations that came up where you grasped something important about what joy is? Try to briefly describe the event and try not to judge or draw conclusions—What happened?

When both have shared their stories we might ask:

Could you give each event a suitable name?

Next, we will invite Margot and Melody to choose one of the stories:

Looking at these experiences of joy, which one intrigues you the most? Which event would you like to delve deeper into to know more about what joy is, and what are your reasons for that?

You chose "hilltop", and it is a good event for exploring what joy might be in more depth. We might be quick to judge the meaning of things in a generic way, but this is also an exercise in stepping back, holding back, wondering and trying to see anew, as for the first time. Could you Margot describe the situation before joy manifested itself—what happened when joyJoy manifested itself—and what had changed after joyJoy manifested itself? As you talk through it, please try to describe bodily sensations and all the senses (Merleau-Ponty, 1962)?

Thank you. Now Melody, and can I ask you what we need to see before our eyes, and to know, to really be able to live ourselves into the situation and understand?

Fine, thank you again, I think we have a clearer and richer picture now.

Step 3: Explore and Find the Essential Characteristics of the Phenomena in the Narrative

The next step in the exploration is to find key characteristics of the phenomena, between the story and the chosen theme:

I will try to recapitulate the event now and correct me if I miss out on something. Exactly where in this sequence of events and this story do you both think joy stands out most clearly? Where does "joy" show itself, and make itself manifest? Choose two specific points, words or events where you feel joy "jumps out" and becomes recognizable and clear for you, and try to explain how. I will also choose my "defining moments" from the story.

Now we have six elements or sentences where we think joy manifests itself in this story. Philosophical inquiry can be said to be the road travelled from asking a question to answering it, and testing the answer. A good philosophical question has some characteristics that lays out a path: it is firstly grounding, in the sense of experientially real, that is we can encounter and experience the thing we are exploring. Secondly it is deeply personal, it can only be experienced by a person, through their specific way of being, sensing and seeing things. Thirdly, it is common for us as humans, it is not absolutely idiosyncratic but says something of interest and relevance to all of us. And fourthly, there are no clear-cut answers we can underscore, it opens up for wonder, and is open ended in that it manifests its value through the test of practice in everyday life.

The two first characteristics are met, what we explore is possible to experience, and it is a deeply personal experience Margot is sharing with us to help us understand. What about the third characteristic, is it common for us as human beings? Can we test this by trying to make the defining moments more universal? Let us try to make each of the six defining moments into the continuation of the sentence "Joy is…", and more, try to make the sentence strive to be true for all people, at all times, everywhere! I will write the sentences down.

Now we have six good sentences describing the central characteristics of what joy is. Can we rate them, from most important to least? Vote your number one, two and three, and give us your reasons.

Step 4: Explore and Challenge What We Find

So, these hierarchical characteristics describing what joy is, does and means, do they have any bearing on the events you shared, and gave names initially? Do they clarify or hide your experience of joy in those instances? Is anything too much, missing, or feels off?

Now we have tested the characteristics on your other experiences, and also some of mine, and give or take a little we have found some central characteristics that are actually useful in explaining what joy is, does and might mean in wildly different events that are important, not just for the one experiencing the event we have explored, but for both of you!

Step 5: Strengthening What We Find in Everyday Life and Relationship

I think you have worked forth something akin to being true, and I think your defining characteristics are beautiful. Have we also worked out something useful? Could these characteristics form your working hypothesis for what to strengthen in everyday life, to strengthen your community going forward?

Could you make these characteristics present in your daily life, and try to take notice of what you would like to keep going and maybe strengthen in your situation, and what you would like to change, to move you both towards experiencing more joy?

What do you both need to happen, to do, that the other does, that other people do, to make each of these characteristics more influential in your everyday life? Can we make a little "action plan" on each of the characteristics for the next small steps to take, and see if that gets us somewhere? Shall we write it down?

When we have explored an existential theme, it is a good idea to check out the attendees' experience:

So, in this exploration, what have you become aware of? Was anything important? What are your takeaways? How was it overall, being you, with us, working with these themes, in this way?

Thank you for useful feedback. I want to thank you for this exploration and your openness!

Alternative Themes to Explore

The steps above are formally indicative and could be applied to other existential themes already present in our example, or other themes Margot and Melody became aware of during the community of inquiry that they might want to explore further.

They might have found it useful to explore their lifeworlds. To clarify "what world are you living in, what is your take at what kind of place this is?", as a basis for being "on the same page" or knowing when they are not, could be helpful (Clifton et al., 2019).

We could have explored the relation between freedom and responsibility: what is freedom, what limits freedom, what is responsibility, and what is a good choice? To build acceptance for differences, and find common ground (Sartre, 2020).

We could have explored values. What is important/gives meaning? Where are you on the continuum between meaning and meaninglessness, meaning-making and meaning-receiving? Where do you want to be, what do you need to see happening to get there (Frankl, 2011)?

We could explore conflict, disconnection, frustration, fights, being annoyed for little things, loneliness and wanting to share experience, knowing that important values are at stake but that "…where danger is, grows the saving power also" (Heidegger, 1977).

We could explore identity-loneliness-attachment, to understand the basis for creating a common life and sharing experience and be closer. What does it mean to be me, with you? What does it mean to relate, to be a couple? When were we who we want to be, where are we now, and where do we want to be? How can we get there (Buber, 2010)?

We could explore authenticity and identity, through experiences of really owning your world, identity and meaning. What does it mean to be me? Exploring an event where I grasped something important (Gadamer, 2003).

We could explore uncertainty/epistemology. There are things we know we know, things we know we don't know and things we don't even know we don't know. Can we venture from order to chaos and back to widen our known world, together (Campbell, 2008)?

We could explore what vulnerability in a limited life means by exploring an event where they grasped something important about what, in the face of adversity, quality of life entails. What does it mean to be, to be me, and to be going to be sick, and ultimately not be? What is "quality of life" for me, given the limits of existence in relation to unavoidable sickness and death (Heidegger, 2001).

Conclusion What Can Existential Exploration Offer Couples?

"What? More questions? But we wanted answers!" Sometimes authentically asking the question anew is the presupposition for an answer. Asking the "big" questions can reveal "the whole" and let us contextualize the answers we already live out in "the parts" and situations of everyday life. Asking them together lets us explore and evaluate whether the answers we live by still fit the big picture and whether they are beneficial to our overall quality of life.

The answers are not "given" or "found" in therapy but an experiential working hypothesis on what might have value in itself despite "all" that challenge it can be construed and tested and lived out in everyday life. Frankl's statement that "he who has a why to live for can bear with almost any how" (Frankl, 2011), might be too bold, yet still retain some truth. Authentically searching for a common working hypothesis to test, and having experienced a way of relating and exploring that knows that it does not know, but wonders, and exploring shared values and practices, a way of cooperating that feels meaningful might come in handy when life confronts us with the unsolvable questions and dilemmas it does, for all of us.

In this process the crumbs on the floor might find their place in the bigger picture, not only as a stumbling stone, but as a clue for finding a way.

We hope we have shown a feasible example of doing existential inquiry to help couples. Margot and Melody wanted to communicate better, avoid conflicts, solve issues, reverse dissolving tendencies and be closer, and we hope we have pointed to one way of moving towards where they want to be. Furthermore, we hope that you have become curious about how to venture forth into the unknowns of existential themes and phenomena in your practice in your own way, thus ever more "becoming who you are" (Nietzsche, 2001), not only as a therapist, but as you.

References

Binder, P.-E. (2020). *Eksistensiell psykologi* [Existential psychology]. Fagbokforlaget.

Buber, M. (2010). *I and Thou*. Martino Fine Books.

Campbell, J. (2008). *The hero with a thousand faces*. New World Library.

Clifton, J. D. W., Baker, J. D., Park, C. L., Yaden, D. B., Clifton, A. B. W., Terni, P., Miller, J. L., Zeng, G., Giorgi, S., Schwartz, H. A., & Seligman, M. E. P. (2019). Primal world beliefs. *Psychological Assessment, 31(1), 82–99*.

Frankl, V. E. (2011). Man's search for meaning : the classic tribute to hope from the Holocaust (New ed., pp. XXVI, 147). Rider.

Gadamer, H.-G. (2003). *Truth and method*. Continuum.

Garrison, D. R. (2015). *Thinking collaboratively: Learning in a community of inquiry*. Routledge.

Hansen, F.-T. (2008). *At stå i det åbne: dannelse gennem filosofisk undren og nærvær* [Standing in the open: Formation through philosophical wonder and presence]. Hans Reitzel.

Hansen, F.-T. (2015). The call and practice of wonder: How to evoke a Socratic Community of wonder in professional settings. In M. N. Weiss (Ed.), *The Socratic handbook*. LIT Verlag.

Heidegger, M. (1977). *The question concerning technology*. Garland Publishing.

Heidegger, M. (2001). *Being and time*. Blackwell Publishers Ltd.

Merleau-Ponty, M. (1962). *Phenomenology of perception*. Routledge.

Nelson, L. (1922). The Socratic Method. https://www.friesian.com/method.htm

Nietzsche, F. (2001). *The gay science*. Cambridge University Press.

Norwegian Directorate of Health [Helsedirektoratet]. (2016). *Gode liv i Norge. Utredning om måling av befolkningens livskvalitet* [A good life in Norway. A review of measurement of the population's quality of life].

Sartre, J.-P. (2020). *Being and nothingness*. Routledge.

Skjervheim, H. (1996). *Participant and spectator, selected essays*. The Department of Philosophy.

Solvoll, B.-A. & Lindseth, A. (2016). The issue of being touched. *Medicine, health care, and philosophy. 19. 10.1007/s11019-015-9682-1.*

Thorsted, A. C., & Hansen, F. T. (2022). *At Tænke med hjertet. En grundbog i eksistensiel praksisfænomenologi* [Thinking with the heart. A primer in existential practice phenomenology]. Klim.

van Deurzen, E., & Arnold-Baker, C. (2018). *Existential therapy. Distinctive features*. Routledge.

Yalom, I. D. (1980). *Existential therapy*. Basic Books.

9

Should I Stay, or Should I Go? Rethinking Identity and the Experience of Migration as a Systemic Dialogue in Therapy

Nicoletta Businaro, Leandra Perrotta, and Jennifer Aramini

Moving to another country is a challenging life transition which requires psychological, social and cultural accommodations. Due to the growth of migration flows, an increasing number of studies have explored different aspects of the migration process. Individual (e.g., personality and motivation), interpersonal (e.g., family dynamics and social network) and cultural factors (e.g., ethnic background) have been identified as strictly interrelated and highly significant in explaining adaptation to a new country (Bucher-Maluschke et al., 2017; Tabor & Milfont, 2011). When persons move abroad, they need to rethink

N. Businaro (✉)
VID Specialized University, Oslo, Norway
e-mail: Nicoletta.businaro@vid.no

L. Perrotta • J. Aramini
Oslo, Norway
e-mail: leandra@face2face-therapy.com

© The Author(s), under exclusive license to Springer Nature Switzerland AG 2023   **131**
T. Grover et al. (eds.), *New Horizons in Systemic Practice with Adults*, Palgrave Texts in Counselling and Psychotherapy, https://doi.org/10.1007/978-3-031-30526-9_9

their own identity, to experience a sense of continuity in their life, and a feeling of belonging. The therapeutic context is a possible window onto how people deal with these processes and hopefully offers a time and space to work them through.

Therapy with migrants has both theoretical and practical implications (see Krause, 2012, 2018). According to a systemic approach, therapist and clients co-construct a safe frame where different issues relating (directly and indirectly) to migration can be processed. Together they endeavour to reflect over possible challenges, stressful experiences, unmet expectations, dreams and disillusions. They strive to find new meanings and purpose. Therapist and client are involved in a dialogue on each other's similarities and differences (Rober & De Haene, 2014). The dialogical and emotional connection which characterizes the therapeutic relationship (Bertrando, 2007, 2015) inevitably shapes the identity of both therapist and client. The client learns from the therapist and the therapist learns from the client. Both explore, negotiate and rethink their identity in a systemic dialogue (Hatcher et al., 2012).

Based on these premises, the present chapter has two objectives which are interrelated. First, it aims to discuss issues which can be relevant in the therapeutic setting when the therapist meets clients who have migrated[1] to a new country. Themes, collected by the authors in therapy conversations, are identified and highlighted in the clinical vignettes. Secondly, the authors reflect on what happens in the relationship between therapist and client when they have both migrated from the same country or when the therapist shares the same country of origin as one partner in a culturally diverse couple. Specifically, this part will focus on how the identities of therapist and client intersect, and how possible biases and beliefs, resonance, expectations and common cultural assumptions can be beneficial or limiting for therapeutic aims.

To grasp the complexity of the therapist-client relationship, we adopt a systemic perspective at different levels of analysis: the relationship between macro-micro systems (cultural and individual level), the relationship between therapist and client, and the relationship between different aspects of the self.

---

[1] In this chapter we refer to voluntary migration, and not forced migration (e.g., refugees), which implies specific social and psychological processes.

The Subtle Layers of the Migration Process

I never thought I would move to Norway. If someone had told me that one day I would wake up in the dark, cold, and snowy Norwegian winter, I'd have laughed.

But I met him. We are raising our children in the dark, cold, and snowy Norwegian winter, but we also enjoy the warm and shining sun in the spring and summer.

Do I sometimes think about moving back to Italy? I suppose that in my mind and in my heart, there will always be this thought buzzing. I miss my family and close friends very much. But if I think about the quality of life that I experience here, and about the possibilities the future holds for my children, I won't move back (for now!).—(Nicoletta, therapist)

When I first moved here, I fell in love with Norway. It was thrilling! I felt like I was on a grand adventure. My honeymoon with Norway, however, was soon over. My friends had told me about culture shock, but I didn't imagine I would feel like a fish out of water. How could I deal with the culture without the shock? It is a roller coaster of emotions. Sometimes I am happy, sometimes I am sad and frustrated.

Should I stay in Norway? Should I go back to Italy?—(Renata, client)

The two quotes above highlight different and significant aspects involved in the process of migration and illustrate some of the issues this chapter focuses on. We have decided to begin this chapter by spotlighting the main characters, the therapist and the client, who are both migrants, and explore the imaginable connections between them.

Before entering the discourse about advantages and possible limitations of this unique therapeutic relationship, we shall broaden our perspective to define the context in which the encounter between therapist and client takes place.

The term migration refers to the movement of people from one geographical place to another. It is a natural phenomenon that has always taken place, but it has changed and increased, both quantitatively and qualitatively.[2] In Europe the number of people moving to another

---

[2] Cfr. https://worldmigrationreport.iom.int/wmr-2022-interactive/.

country has substantially increased in the last twenty years, due to several factors such as international, political and economic policies, an increasing accessibility to travel, and expanding social networks of family and friends. Among the reasons motivating a person to move to another country, are opportunities for a better quality of life, higher income, reuniting the family and political stability. If in earlier times, the migration process mainly involved adults, nowadays younger people are the ones who most frequently take this decision. Furthermore, there is an increasingly substantial migration of skilled and highly educated young adults, a phenomenon referred to as the "brain drain".

There is a conspicuous debate about which terms are more appropriate to use when it comes to migration. In this chapter we use the term "migration" to refer to the "process of migration", based on two main reasons. First, as Tabor and Milfont (2011) pointed out, the term "emigrant" refers to someone leaving their own country of origin to settle in another one, whereas the term "immigrant" indicates the person in relationship to the country they settle in. Immigrants are also emigrants, though not every emigrant will become an immigrant. Therefore, a preferable term is "migrant", which embodies the complexity of the process. From a psychological perspective, migration is a developmental process with its own phases and transitions. The migration change model, developed by Tabor and Milfont (2011), identifies three phases: preparation, moving, and the attempt to achieve psychological adjustment and sociocultural adaptation. The first phase is characterized by an imaginative process. Possibilities are considered, and the idea of migration slowly takes shape. This phase may be accompanied by the desire for self-development, or the wish to accomplish something greater. In the second phase, the possibility of moving is planned, and actively implemented. The last phase is characterized by the arrival in a new country, which can be exciting and full of wonder, as well as a stressful and disorienting experience. In the new environment, the person must make certain choices regarding where to live, how to learn the language and find a job. A more refined and arduous process regards the revision of the migrant's beliefs, values and ideals which need to be integrated into the new cultural system. The migrant must accommodate to new ways of communicating, both linguistically and meta-linguistically, and to understand the workings of the new political system and bureaucracy. The acculturation process challenges the person physically and psychologically. Each person's unique way of coping with the challenges determines their psychological and social wellbeing. Rather than viewing the process of acculturation in a linear way, it is worthwhile recognizing and appreciating the ongoing fluidity of this process. Even when a migrant settles down, they face a continuous decision-making process regarding the choice to stay, return or move to another country. In this sense, the migration process begins before the act of relocation and continues indefinitely thereafter.

Secondly, the emphasis that this is a process implies that we need to adopt a broader perspective to grasp the complexity. The individual is viewed in relation to the social and cultural context, which connects to the existing reference system. Migration is an individual and family transition, in time and space, which presupposes individual, social and cultural accommodations (Falicov, 2016). In the life cycle of a family, migration is considered a non-normative event. It can occur unexpectedly, it is not experienced by all families, and it is rarely imagined in the original plan of life (McGoldrick et al., 2005). As a non-normative event, it can lead to the opportunity of cultivating a richer and more creative life, acquiring a better education and establishing new relationships. It can also be potentially distressing. Even when migration involves one family member only, the whole family system, as well as the future generations, is affected by this event. The migration story is integrated into the family narrative, and the repercussions have transgenerational implications. The migrant's life experience can impact the identity of the descendants and forge the lenses through which they see the world.

The separation process experienced in migration often leads to a sense of loss and longing of family, friends and loved ones. As time goes by, migrants can even experience the loss of fluency in their native language. Nostalgia, and a partial understanding of social and cultural norms, can reinforce the sense of not belonging. The migrant may find themselves without an adequate job, and without the support of the social system of which they used to be a part. Skills and competencies which were relevant in the country of origin (such as education or professional experience) may not be recognized in the new country. Most of the "known" is replaced by the "unknown". The migrant may need to rethink and recontextualize their identity to come to terms with the loss of certain aspects of their culture of origin and must learn to deal with the perception of discontinuity in the new social reality. Migration poses the challenge of becoming proficient with uncomfortable emotions, dealing with a sense of unease and loneliness, gaining an understanding of the new practical and ideological realities, and learning how to grasp possible opportunities for a satisfying life.

The migration process embodies a sense of loss and gain for the person who leaves, and the family in the home country is often filled with expectations and fantasies about the opportunities for their family member abroad. Attempting to fulfil these expectations may easily become a burden for the migrant.

The therapist accesses the intricacy of all these processes to find resources to help the client rebound from crisis and cultivate hope. Envisioning migration in all its complexity, as an ongoing and ambivalent process, requires therapists to adopt a systemic perspective for the purposes of assessment, intervention and prevention. A systemic perspective considers the physical and emotional relations of the client with the new environment, place of origin, family and friends at home, with the therapist and with themselves.

What Happens in the Therapy Room When Both Therapist and Client Are Migrants?

Therapist and client co-create a safe space to reflect on the opportunities, challenges and expectations relating to the process of migration. They strive to develop a new sense of meaning and purpose, and to find a red thread which can establish a sense of continuity between the past life in their country of origin and life in the present and future. As Italian psychotherapists who have chosen to settle down in Norway, we find ourselves meeting with Italian individual clients, and culturally diverse couples living in Norway, of which one of the partners is Italian. Below, we explore some of the issues we experience as recurring in our conversations. These issues include the stories of individuals, families, several families, of society and of one or more cultures.

Intergenerational Implications and Cultural Assumptions

Roberto is an Italian man who has been living in Norway for twelve years. His therapeutic request is to understand the frustration he feels. Although he claims to have adjusted to Norway quite well, certain experiences clash with his idea of what is adequate, especially regarding the education of his children. Roberto has two sons, and during a session, he complains about the school system in Norway. He is extremely vocal about how children are taught to write and says to Nicoletta (the therapist), "You know how schools are in Italy. Teachers there are much more capable at teaching children how to write". Nicoletta invites him to explain what teachers do in Norway, and what teachers do in Italy (based on his experience) and to unpack his reasoning. It becomes increasingly evident that his complaints are in reality, concerns. Roberto is worried that his two sons will not learn to write neatly and beautifully. Calligraphy holds a special meaning because it represents discipline, a highly regarded value for him. Nicoletta probes further and asks, "does this mean you are worried that your children will not learn discipline? Does it mean you are concerned they will not learn the same values you were taught in Italy?" This leads to a series of reflections regarding the intergenerational values Roberto wishes to transmit to his sons and their cultural significance.

This example proposes a relevant theme: the need as a parent to reflect on the values he wishes to transmit to his children, and what he believes is important for them to learn. This is culturally related. The father grew up in a different context to that in which the children are being raised, and must reconcile the values he holds, with those he is experiencing in Norway, the country he has settled in. Roberto's concerns and frustration derive from a possible conflict of values that are triggered by a specific behaviour (learning to write at school) but refer to something much broader (discipline and general values). If the therapist had simply validated the client's concerns, she would have missed reflecting on Roberto's implicit assumption that sharing the same Italian heritage meant possessing similar categories of conceptual knowledge. The client assumed that the therapist understood Italian norms, and held similar values and beliefs, simply because they were both Italian. A background of knowledge is undoubtedly shared, but the experience of being Italian can be quite diverse. Despite sharing the same country of origin, therapist and client may have little in common despite a broad categorical understanding of the country's school policies and relating values. The "not-knowing" position (Anderson & Goolishian, 1992) where the therapist does not assume to know what the person is referring to, but maintains a genuine interest, and asks to elaborate, helps the client to reflect on the meaning of his personal experience and brings awareness to his socially constructed view of the world.

Rethinking Identity: Reframing and Self-disclosure

Federico, a middle-aged man, seeks therapy after having separated from his spouse. He had moved from Italy to be with his pregnant wife. He finds himself living far away from his family and friends. He finds it difficult to learn the Norwegian language and to find a job which is suitable to his experience and education. He feels he is losing his sense of self and wonders what he is doing in Norway. He feels life is meaningless and seems to question everything. Jennifer (the therapist) listens carefully and validates the anger and sadness he feels. The therapist shares with him about her personal experience of moving to Norway, focusing on the challenges she experienced, as she carefully redirects the dialogue towards the possibilities and choices available to Federico (such as searching for satisfying professional opportunities).

Moving to another country as an adult requires facing certain challenges, such as learning a new language and getting a job. This often happens without the support of family and close friends. The possible difficulties can create self-limiting beliefs about one's abilities and lead to questioning life in the new country, as well as one's purpose in life. This is even more remarkable when his wife, his only connection (and possible motivation) to stay in the new country, is no longer present in Federico's life. When struggling, it is common to feel alone. The therapist encourages the client to reframe his experience, brings in new perspectives and helps him to short circuit his narrative. She normalizes the client's experience and shares anecdotes about her own challenges during the migration process. She facilitates the understanding that other people (even therapists) can go through similar predicaments. Honest and authentic self-disclosure (Hedges, 2010) helps the client not to feel judged and allows him to voice his pain. Emotional closeness is needed to reflect on himself, his unmet needs and expectations, and how to rethink his identity in a new cultural and social context. The therapist chooses to share some of her own experiences regarding migration to acknowledge and validate the emotions of the client and to guide him to explore new possibilities. In a therapeutic process, the change in perspective from "I don't know who I am, I don't know what to do" to "is there something I can do?" reflects an emotional transformation from a sense of loss and confusion to a sentiment of hope.

Musings About "Home"

> Amanda is a 13-year-old girl who starts her first session by talking about her life and crying, "I don't know where to live. I don't like it here in Norway and I don't like it in Italy. I feel lost. I don't know where home is". Her mother does not know how to help her teenage daughter and does not understand why she is progressively shutting the world out. She spends most of her time alone in her room, has very few friends and is often sad and irritable. Mother and daughter come from a small village in the South of Italy and moved to Norway five years ago, after the mother received an excellent job offer. Amanda was eight when they moved and her encounter with Norway had seemed quite positive at the time. Her mother describes how Amanda adjusted to school quite readily, thanks to learning the Norwegian language quickly and fluently. On the one hand, the mother highlights the positive aspects of the Norwegian lifestyle, and Amanda's skills, which allow her to have a satisfying life in Norway; on the other hand, Amanda refers to a sense of sadness and loneliness derived from not feeling at home. Amanda does not feel she belongs, either in Norway or in Italy. Nicoletta (the therapist), guides Amanda to reflect on the meaning of "home" and tries to encourage an empathic sharing between mother and daughter.

This vignette exemplifies the complexity of the sense of belonging. Home is a physical and symbolic point of reference. When we find ourselves disoriented, we look for home. Amanda is in a critical developmental phase for the formation of her identity. As an adolescent, it is crucial to find her reference points and a sense of belonging. Belonging is facilitated and hindered by people and experiences which dynamically interact with the individual's identity (Allen et al., 2021). Identity and belonging are strictly intertwined. We understand who we are and who we are not, through our relationship to others and to the world. Migration to another country also requires moving to a new home, both practically and psychologically. The developmental phase of adolescence, as well as the process of migration, challenges Amanda's sense of belonging. Most people have a deep need to feel a sense of belonging, characterized as a positive and reciprocal connection with other people, places or experiences. When the sense of belonging wanes, people can suffer from social isolation, loneliness and a lack of connection to others. Where is home? This is a question which awakens deep feelings in the therapist as she reflects on what home is and where home is. In the therapeutic process, the therapist relives her own experience of separation from her Italian home and the creation of a new Norwegian home. The therapist relies on her own personal experience to help Amanda orient herself in her jumble of thoughts and feelings, by asking her questions the therapist has already asked herself. Although Amanda and her therapist find themselves in two different stages of life (adolescent and adult), the issue of belonging is central and accentuated in the migration process.

Conflict of Loyalty: Should I Stay, or Should I Go?

Arianna, an Italian woman in her 30s, met Arne while he was doing his Erasmus in Italy. They fell in love and got married. They settled down in Arianna's hometown and had two young children. Arne had a promising career and had recently received a prestigious job opportunity back home in Norway. Arianna's parents were devastated by their decision to move away. They were scared their grandchildren would not learn to speak Italian, that they would miss seeing them grow up, and ultimately lose their relationship with them. Arianna was excited about living in Norway, but after her move, she started to feel a lot of pressure and a strong sense of obligation to her family of origin. Her loyalty was torn between her parents, who were getting older, her husband's wish to have a successful career in Norway, and the duty to provide her children with a care-free life in a country she described as "safe and easy". Arianna and Arne requested couples therapy because she was plagued with a sense of guilt. She had started to suffer from migraines with increasing intensity, precipitated by her growing anxiety. Her stress was impacting their relationship, and the tension between them was growing. She found herself blaming her husband, feeling resentful, and questioning the decision to move, she had been so eager to comply with, only recently. She was tormented by her conflict, and when presenting her frustration in the session, Arianna expected Leandra (the therapist) to share and support her view that Italian families demanded a strong sense of loyalty and spirit of sacrifice from their members. Arianna asks the therapist to convey this belief to her Norwegian husband: "you are Italian. Please explain to Arne how important loyalty to family is". Arianna tries to draw the therapist in even further by asking her if her parents are still alive and does she not feel guilty knowing they are growing old without her presence and support. The therapist carefully brings awareness to this dynamic and points out Arianna's conflict of loyalty.

Arianna is feeling disoriented, angry, and her unease is expressed with psychosomatic symptoms. The body speaks louder than words. Arianna's experience exemplifies what is defined as "invisible loyalty" in transgenerational family therapy (Böszörményi-Nagy, 1984). The sense of loyalty Arianna feels towards her family of origin conflicts with her sense of loyalty towards her husband and her children and with the idea of raising her children in a country perceived as safe. The challenge of finding adequate and satisfying ways of maintaining a relationship with her family of origin, as well as a relationship with her new family, is natural in the cycle of life. When a person migrates, the physical and geographical distance from one's family of origin is even more evident. Arianna's parents are worried that physical distance will inevitably translate into emotional distance. Arianna's parents, husband and children all expect loyalty from her. Arianna somatises the tensions dictated by the multiple demands of loyalty towards her and her own sense of loyalty to her family. Arianna's attempt at triangulating the therapist, based on the implicit assumption that they share similar values and beliefs because they are both Italian, risks contaminating the trust and therapeutic alliance with Arne, who is starting to feel excluded, misunderstood, and feels his wife is trying to manipulate the therapist. Holding the space so that both partners can feel seen and validated takes a lot of focus and energy, and requires the therapist to be aware of her own ambivalent feelings about having left her family in Italy.

Resources and Traps Behind a Common Cultural Origin

When examining the nuts and bolts of working within an intercultural framework, most of the literature considers situations in which therapist and migrant come from different countries and investigates similarities and differences revolving around culture when brought to the therapeutic space (see Ertl et al., 2019). Less attention has been drawn to the implications concerning the encounter between therapist and client, when both are migrants and both come from the same country. It is an interesting and specific situation, considering that both have experienced the process of migration. Our questions and interest focus on how the therapist can use their own experience of migration to attune to the client, and how it can affect their understanding.

When therapist and client have both migrated from the same country of origin, it is highly probable that both view that experience as a connection. Cultural identity becomes predominant, and it can be a resource as well as a possible trap for the therapeutic process.

When first contacting us, clients often point out that their choice of therapist is based on their assumption of a shared, cultural origin. Italians choose Italians because they are Italian. It is not surprising that in a foreign country, in which clients might feel disempowered and perceive a lesser mastery of their surroundings, they would choose someone whom they feel they can relate to, and by whom they imagine they would feel understood. This can increase the therapist's sense of self-efficacy and enhance the emotional connection and rapport with the client. A similar cultural background may foster a sense of likeness, as some theories of social psychology posit (Cabral & Smith, 2011). More than the notion of culture, however, it is the notion of similarity that is worthwhile focusing on. The feeling of being alike can provide credibility, trust, a sense of ease and of understanding in the client, in relation to the therapist (Ames, 2004). The sense of similarity can spark a sense of communal belonging, reinforce the therapeutic alliance and facilitate a collaborative setting.

Resonance can be a powerful dynamic when the client shares life stories which are similar to those experienced by the therapist. The similarity can contribute to an increased sense of empathy and emotional closeness. Hedges (2010) reflects on how the therapist can share feelings, beliefs, and experiences from their personal life to create connection, improve rapport and further the therapeutic process.

The therapist, however, must be mindful about not colluding with the client and ensure the possibility of a reflective space. It is crucial to intuit when to shed light on the resonance to help the client feel less alone, and conversely, to understand when resonance can become a trap and possibly damage the therapeutic process. The therapist must always assess the rationale for self-disclosure, the possible impact it might have on the client, and question if the process is motivated by the intention to deepen the relationship with the client and enhance a feeling of availability and shared vulnerability.

Resonance can be limiting when the therapist's own migration experience has not been completely processed. This can lead the therapist to project their own unfinished business on the client and make assumptions based on their own unresolved issues (Aponte, 2022). Resonance can easily lead the therapist into the terrain of the implicit. It is therefore crucial to develop the curiosity to explore what seems to be known and familiar. This implies self-reflexivity whereby the therapist reflects and becomes aware of their own cognitive and emotional processes.

The reflexive position can be supported and stimulated in supervision. The relevance of supervision is essential in the development of a competent therapist. It is within the context of supervision that the therapist can share beliefs, biases, emotionally draining experiences, resources and traps relating to the therapeutic process with the client. The therapist can reflect on their own unfinished business and ethical doubts. Supervision should give the therapist opportunities for theoretical and practical learning, for personal and professional development and for self-care. The relationship between supervisee and supervisor can provide the confidential environment for reflexivity, safety, and care the therapist may need. During supervision the therapist can learn new skills and ways to deal with clients and find emotional support (Sheehan, 2016; Vetere & Sheehan, 2017).

Concluding Thoughts

The clinical vignettes exemplify the complexity of working in an intercultural setting. A systemic perspective allows us to grasp the dynamics between client and therapist, as well as their internal processes, in relation to a broader cultural framework. The issues which emerge in a therapeutic process with migrants are often explicitly tied to existential questions: Who am I? Where do I belong? What values do I believe in, and what do I want to transmit to my children? Where is home? What is my sense of purpose? Am I loyal to my family of origin or to my new family? (See Chaps. 6 and 8 for a broader discussion on existential issues.)

Culture informs and shapes our identity, and when we adapt to a new cultural environment, we need to rethink, redefine and recontextualize our identity. These processes can strengthen the therapeutic alliance when both therapist and client have experienced migration. Shared cultural identity can enhance trust and foster a sense of increased understanding of the client. Implicit assumptions and biases, however, must always be considered, and the risk of triangulation, when working with culturally diverse couples, must be held in awareness. Each client can awaken memories, experiences, wounds, pains and dreams in the therapist. It is how the therapist deals with the resonance in meeting the other person, that is the heart of therapy (Elkaïm, 1997).

It is vital to reflect on how close we can allow ourselves to be to the client, without invading their personal space, and without colouring their stories with our stories. It is relevant to recognize the processes we share with the client, what differentiates us, and at the same time, recognize and appreciate the uniqueness of each person in the therapeutic process.

References

Allen, K.-A., Kern, M. L., Rozek, C. S., McInereney, D., & Slavich, G. M. (2021). Belonging: A review of conceptual issues, an integrative framework, and directions for future research. *Australian Journal of Psychology, 73*(1), 87–102. https://doi.org/10.1080/00049530.2021.1883409

Ames, D. (2004). Strategies for social inference: A similarity contingency model of projection and stereotyping in attribute prevalence estimates. *Journal of Personality and Social Psychology, 87*, 573–585. https://doi.org/10.1037/0022-3514.87.5.573

Anderson, H., & Goolishian, H. (1992). The client is the expert: A not-knowing approach to therapy. In S. McNamee & K. J. Gergen (Eds.), *Therapy as social construction* (pp. 25–39). Sage Publications.

Aponte, H. J. (2022). The soul of therapy: The therapist's use of self in the therapeutic relationship. *Contemporary Family Therapy, 44*, 136–143. https://doi.org/10.1007/s10591-021-09614-5

Bertrando, P. (2007). *Dialogical therapist: Dialogue in systemic practice.* Karnac Books.

Bertrando, P. (2015). *Emotions and the therapist: A systemic-dialogical approach.* Karnac Books.

Böszörményi-Nagy, I. (1984). *Invisible loyalties.* Routledge.

Bucher-Maluschke, J., Gondim, M. D. F., & Pedroso, J. D. S. (2017). The effects of migration on family relationships: Case studies. *International Journal of Migration, Health and Social Care, 13*(2), 198–206. https://doi.org/10.1108/IJMHSC-05-2015-0016

Cabral, R. R., & Smith, T. B. (2011). Racial/ethnic matching of clients and therapists in mental health services: A meta-analytic review of preferences, perceptions, and outcomes. *Journal of Counseling Psychology, 58*, 537–554. https://doi.org/10.1037/a0025266

Elkaïm, M. (1997). *If you love me, don't love me: Undoing reciprocal double binds and other methods of change in couple and family therapy.* Basic Books.

Ertl, M. M., Mann-Saumier, M., Martin, R. A., Graves, D. F., & Altarriba, J. (2019). The impossibility of client–therapist "Match": Implications and future directions for multicultural competency. *Journal of Mental Health Counseling, 41*(4), 312–326. https://doi.org/10.17744/mehc.41.4.03

Falicov, C. J. (2016). Migration and the family life cycle, Chapter 12. In M. McGoldrick, N. Garcia-Preto, & B. Carter (Eds.), *The expanded family life cycle: Individual, family and social perspectives* (5th ed.). Allyn & Bacon.

Hatcher, S. L., Kipper-Smith, A., Waddell, M., Uhe, M., West, J. S., Boothe, J. H., Frye, J. M., Tighe, K., Usselman, K. L., & Gingras, P. (2012). What therapists learn from psychotherapy. *The Qualitative Report, 17*, 1–21. https://doi.org/10.46743/2160-3715/2012.1702

Hedges, F. (2010). *Reflexivity in therapeutic practice*. Palgrave Macmillan.

Krause, I.-B. (2012). *Culture and reflexivity in systemic psychotherapy: Mutual perspectives*. Karnac Books.

Krause, I.-B. (2018). *Culture and system in family therapy*. Taylor & Francis.

McGoldrick, M., Giordano, J., & Garcia-Preto, N. (Eds.). (2005). *Ethnicity and family therapy* (3rd ed.). The Guilford Press.

Rober, P., & De Haene, L. (2014). Intercultural therapy and the limitations of a cultural competency framework: About cultural differences, universalities and the unresolvable tensions between them. *Journal of Family Therapy, 36*(Suppl. 1), 3–20. https://doi.org/10.1111/1467-6427.12009

Sheehan, J. (2016). Self and world: Narrating experience in the supervisor/supervisee relationship. In I. A. Vetere & P. Stratton (Eds.), *Interacting selves. Systemic solutions for personal and professional development in counselling and psychotherapy* (pp. 109–129). Routledge.

Tabor, A. S., & Milfont, T. L. (2011). Migration change model: Exploring the process of migration on a psychological level. *International Journal of Intercultural Relations, 35*, 818–832. https://doi.org/10.1016/j.ijintrel.2010.11.013

Vetere, A., & Sheehan, J. (Eds.). (2017). *Supervision of family therapy and systemic practice*. Springer.

10

If We Only Met Once? A Talk with Five Single Session Orientated Therapists

Sigurd Riste Andersen

Introduction

Single session therapy (SST) has since its first description in 1990 grown in influence (see Dryden, 2019; Hoyt et al., 2018; Talmon, 1990; Söderquist, 2020; Söderquist, 2023; Young & Rycroft, 2012; Young & Rycroft, 2020; Bloom, 2001; Campbell, 2012). Single session therapy, and the thinking (Hoyt et al., 2020) underlying it, challenges the idea that therapy must involve many sessions. Research suggests that many clients attend only one, yet find this one session helpful. If this research is accepted, there are significant opportunities to harness the possibility that change, even significant change, can happen as a result of one or a few sessions, especially if we embrace the power of *here and now*. This chapter will describe *what* SST is by presenting the experiences of five therapists who use SST with families and couples.

S. R. Andersen (✉)
VID Specialized University, Oslo, Norway
e-mail: Sigurd.andersen@vid.no

© The Author(s), under exclusive license to Springer Nature Switzerland AG 2023   **147**
T. Grover et al. (eds.), *New Horizons in Systemic Practice with Adults*, Palgrave Texts in
Counselling and Psychotherapy, https://doi.org/10.1007/978-3-031-30526-9_10

Single session therapy is opening new horizons in systemic psychotherapy and is creating frameworks that aim to create processes that are client led and designed to help families to be active in dealing with problems. This perspective is co-creative which relieves the therapists from having to adopt an expert-position in therapy. SST might be used with families dealing with challenges such as violence or trauma, but with the possibility of the family needing a longer process of therapy (Campbell, 2012; Doorn & Sweeney, 2019; Le Gros et al., 2019; O'Neill, 2017; Rose et al., 2003). SST is not a method, nor a manual, but is a framework that is flexible for therapists with different styles and approaches to use. Alliance is an important part of any therapeutic process. SST seeks to build relational alliance quickly reinforced with an alliance formed by focusing on what is important for the client, regardless if the client has clear goals for the therapy or not. SST may be considered to be closer to the field of consultation than other therapeutic approaches. Even though the name *Single Session Therapy* might bring expectations of only one session being offered, the idea behind SST is rather to make the most out of every session and the time available and to provide options for further work if the client desires it. This attitude might help everyone involved in being more focused on changes and important moments in the session. This chapter is written from a systemic, relational perspective and will describe the use of SST with families and couples respectively. As Martin Söderquist describes it: *the goal is change, whether it happens in one session or seven.*

In my own private therapy practice, I usually mention at the beginning of the first session, "We have this session today, we may schedule more sessions, based on how we work together and your need". As I have written a book chapter on single session thinking with an inter-disciplinary focus earlier (Andersen, 2021), I am somewhat influenced by SST in my own way of working. I do believe different people connect differently to different therapists and approaches and I see SST as an important addition to already established approaches with longer therapeutic processes. I would at the same time take this opportunity to recommend reading the chapter in this very book called *Agape* by Sheehan and Vetere. The chapter describes how long-term relationships in therapy can be important and necessary for people who have suffered from a lack of stability and loving care in their lives. The chapter shows the variety of how therapists work, but also the importance of being open to different needs with the families and couples we meet.

In the process of writing this book chapter I have interviewed five other therapists who are using single session therapy with couples or families. They have all given their acceptance for their contribution and being named in this chapter. The first interview was made with Martin Söderquist, a Swedish psychologist and family therapist who has been working within child and adolescent psychiatry and family counselling. The second interview was with four therapists attached to the Bouverie Centre in Melbourne, Australia: Lynda Moore, Karen Story, Kelly Tsorlinis and Jeff Young, the former director of the Bouverie Centre. The Bouverie Centre has 28 years of experience using SST and has established a wide variety of single session services. The four therapists interviewed are a part of several of these, but in particular *women in prison* (WIP), where therapists meet with women and their close relations before and during the release process from prison, and a virtual walk-in family clinic called *walk in together* (WIT). In my interviews with the therapists, I asked them what parts of a single session therapeutic process they saw as particularly important when working with families and couples. Would there be something that facilitates important moments in therapy, and how may these moments be detected? Is there anything they as therapists do to create such moments? How do they detect significant moments for the family? Is there something in a process that is hard to put into words, like atmosphere, expectations, bodily reactions or ambiance in the session?

As family therapy is a vast field, this chapter aims to be relevant for a diversity of professionals in the systemic field. The descriptions will be relevant not only for therapists who are interested in using SST, but are highly relevant for any psychotherapist with a relational, systemic perspective. I hope the following can make you as a reader curious about your own practice and how you work. As Martin Söderquist describes it, a key to a good alliance with a client is the confidence the therapist shows by being safe in their own subject. This underlines the importance of not adopting a method or frame uncritically, but rather to let one be inspired by a variety of approaches and ideas, as described in numerous chapters in this book series. With that said, I hope you are inspired by the single session attitude and framework and may use this chapter as a way of seeing some of the clinical benefits and important moments that might emerge from adopting a *here-and-now*-way of working. Perhaps single session thinking will resonate with something you already do or inspire you to do something you might want to try.

Therapeutic Findings

The following is a thematic description of what the interviewed therapists and myself see as the most important parts of creating meaningful and important moments in therapy with couples and families, within the frame of SST. The themes follow a chronological order and start with the bigger picture that includes the importance of context and process. The next parts will be about preparation and the beginning of a session, during a session, when the session is coming to an end and the process following a session.

The Bigger Picture

There are several parts of the therapeutic process that are of a more overall nature. This includes the context for the session and descriptions of the process as a whole.

Context and Process

The first theme that emerges from the interviews is the importance of the context. As a systemic therapist it is vital to understand the importance of context as nothing makes sense without a context. Context is hence vital to a fundamental understanding of a phenomenon, and a way of creating meaning and directing our expectations. A clear description of the process of a single session approach will help families understand what to expect and hence will help them feel safe and comfortable. If the family and therapist have an expectation of many sessions, a session will typically end with "see you next Thursday". Feedback from families that attend SST indicates that many couples and families can benefit from just one session. Even though we do not know what people bring with them to the therapy room, Jeff Young describes that we might still be able to describe what a session will look like for the families we meet in SST, more so than in traditional therapy. This is because the SST frame gives us a way of asking "how can I be useful to you?" For many therapists this frame is also a big relief, as it avoids the idea that they must fix every problem the families have. Such an idea might easily become paralyzing or pressuring the therapist in the direction of pushing through changes that the family did not really want. The process of SST may contribute to a feeling of direction for the work. Ironically, Young states, one of the findings in research is that the SST approach can be good for families with complex challenges, because of this focus on what should we try and achieve in this session, right here and now. This questions the idea that complex challenges always need long therapeutic processes. Families facing complex problems may not have the time, space or resources to engage in long-term work either.

Like many therapists, community members assume that therapy will typically be long term. Söderquist describes that many couples ask before the first session if they can book several sessions. He responds by saying that "we will see at the end of the session what you need". Söderquist describes that it does not really matter if the change takes seven sessions or just one; the importance is that it happens. In SST we might get there sooner as we focus so much on the here and now, but we must also keep the door open, in case we need more time and more sessions.

Preparation and the Beginning of a Session

Questionnaires

A part of the process of SST to facilitate change is the use of question-naires or other types of pre-session work. It varies from service to service how this is done and to what extent. A pre-questionnaire might open up the possibility to focus on important themes and acknowledge that people will do work before the session. Learning about the family's process before a session may give useful information to a meeting. Karen Story shares an experience where a teenager was asked by her Mom to fill out a questionnaire before a session. The girl wrote a swear word on the form and then tore the whole paper form into pieces. After the incident, the Mom had taped the form back together and brought this with her to the first session, where Story got the chance to acknowledge the form and ask, "So, based on the form, I can really tell you seem quite angry about coming here". They were then able to use this information to talk about what they could do to make the session useful to the girl and her mother.

The First Hello

The first greeting might also be of great importance to make the most out of a session and create important moments. Martin Söderquist describes that how the therapist greets the client and how the therapist creates safety is vital. He shares an example where a woman that came to a session described afterwards that she immediately knew that the session and process would be good for her. Söderquist believes that the frame of SST might contribute to therapists feeling more confident in their work. The therapeutic method in the session is not decisive, but if the method is anchored in the therapist, the family or couple will sense this security indirectly.

Creating a Belief for Change

An important part of a therapy process, also in SST, is that both the therapist and client should *believe* that change is possible. Söderquist shares an experience where a family comes to therapy: The mother says, "We have been to so many therapy sessions, but nothing ever happens". Söderquist answered the mother by saying, "Ok, so if we can make a change, what would that be?" This opened up a space for the mother to share what they could talk further about. It also created room for other voices in the family. A belief that change is possible in therapy is important to make every encounter count. We do not know for sure if clients will come back for a second session or not and, as Karen Story describes it, we must use the presence and excitement of the here and now. To make the most out of the presence, Söderquist refers to Tom Andersen and describes that it is important to make a change that is recognizable to the family, but at the same time different. We cannot simply say that "you are doing great!" and support the family, but should add something new and something the family has not tried before. This calls for the therapist to be creative and being able to think outside of the box. Kelly Tsorlinis describes that a big part of the flow of SST is *change on steroids*. The therapist should be able to use different systemic approaches, lenses and perspectives in bringing new information into the system. We should strive to help the family to look at what has happened and what needs to be done. We could also talk with the family about what they have not had the chance to see happen yet. How would that look?

During the Session

Collaboration

Many of the interviewed therapists describe the importance of collaboration. Söderquist emphasizes that working together with the family or couple is a key element of SST. It is equally important to be *where the other is* and be concerned with what the family brings into the room. In a meeting with a woman Söderquist met in therapy, she stated early in the session that "I have met Jesus". Söderquist and the woman continued talking about this theme and spent the whole session talking about it. They were building the talk on her language and acknowledging that this was the most important theme for her. Söderquist describes that this itself created golden moments for the woman and reinforced experiences that were of great importance to her. In a session it is important that the therapist tries to start with a clean sheet and an open mind. We do not need to read journals or know more than a name to be curious. We are simply talking about "why are we here today, and what could we do together?" Söderquist also brings forward a story where he met a family that started the session by assuming he had read up on documents from other therapists. "Why haven't you read up on journals and reports", they asked. Söderquist shared his thought on the benefits of meeting the family where they were now, and to avoid reading others opinions about them beforehand. This is in line with what Lynda Moore describes. She thinks that the central task of a session is to work together with the family on what direction they want to go. Feedback from families shows that they value the chance to explore where to go next together with the therapist and hence not being directed by the therapist. Jeff Young adds that finding out what people want and what they might think about it might in itself be a solution in therapy. In the process of letting families describe their problem we can make a choice on how we talk about the problem, says Söderquist. As described in the introduction, it might be tempting for therapists to offer advice or solutions in the session. I would like you as a reader to challenge this idea, and try to reflect on "what can I ask the family to help them to develop a process for dealing with their issues, including after the session?" When the family invites us to dialogue about their problem, it is a key point to talk about problems in a way that gives more room for a different process than the problem saturation. This is also a productive way of talking about the problem—a way of acknowledging the problem, but also giving hope and making room for change. A useful question might be "when this problem has less space, how would it be then?"

Embedded Hope

Söderquist describes the importance of embedded hope. By this we mean the hope that is present, but not explicitly spoken of. As therapists we must be aware of how hope, or a lack of it, may be both a powerful and existential topic. Perhaps should we reflect on whether to address hope as a topic, depending on who we meet and the current situation? People in deep despair or in a period of crisis might not see or feel hope at the time and perhaps would talking explicitly about hope just amplify the feeling of hopelessness. When couples and families speak of problems, there is at the same time always an underlying embedded hope for change, Söderquist claims. As therapists we might bring hope to families and couples through the idea of change being possible. A focus on change will be a contrast to problem-talk that might enlarge the problem. Some examples of questions we might ask are "when we end today, what would you bring with you" or "how would you recognize a small difference towards the situation being better for you?" In sessions we can use less time on information about the problem and focus more on how it would be when the problem is less present. Through a focus on hope and how we talk about the problem we can gain momentum to make changes. This benefits the family we are seeing, Söderquist says.

Creativity in How We Work

As therapists we should try to be flexible, creative and try to stay active in our work. We might use language or different interventions to give input and offer changes. We might also use creativity, sculpting, cards, pictures or a variety of ways of offering something for families. Söderquist describes a couple that came to therapy where it seemed unclear for him whether they wanted to stay together in their marriage or not. He asked them to make a mental picture of holding the problems in one hand and the solutions in the other. He then asked them to have a look at their two hands and feel what they both meant to them. He then asked them, "Which of the two hands feels closest to your heart?" The couple looked at each other and simultaneously answered "separation" and laughed. He asked the couple, "Was this what you came here for today?" "Yes", they answered. "So, we are done for today". Söderquist saw this as an example of how he as a therapist could be creative in transferring bodily sensations or feelings into words. The couple then talked for a few moments on how to deal with the next practicalities before leaving.

Safety and Openness

In therapy sessions in general, and SST in particular it is important to create safety and a non-blaming and not judgemental way of meeting families, Kelly Tsorlinis highlights. This helps families get more out of the session. In her experience, a relational perspective and circular perspectives like triangular questions help to create a *flow* in the talk and engage the family. The therapist should also strive to be open and curious, Söderquist states. The family should not be treated as a number or protocol. You should let them know they are unique. Some questions Söderquist are especially fond of are: "how did you do that", "I haven't thought about that before, how did you get there" and "what did you do to succeed on that?" When we ask questions like this we are interested in the uniqueness of the family and might also contribute in creating pivotal moments. Pivotal moments could be of a quantitative nature, where change happens several times in everyday life, or we could create a qualitative change, an important *here and now* experience. Humour could also contribute to making pivotal moments, Söderquist says. If we create a way of talking about serious themes, but at the same time might have a hint of humour, it is possible to make a stronger connection between everyone in the room. Therapy is a different context from home and the perspective of seeing a situation from the outside might create a meta-view and help us point out the absurdity of the situation or an outside look at oneself. Even though openness, curiousness and humour will not make pivotal moments in itself, they make a good frame for that to happen, Söderquist states.

Towards the End and After a Session

Towards the end of a SST there are several ways of offering interventions for families and couples. This might include reflections, summaries, listening for feedback and for therapists to use a team.

Sharing Reflections

During a session it might be a good idea to share reflections in front of the family. This is described as a common intervention in SST with the aim of creating new paths and helping the family in their process. Lynda Moore describes that through a reflection we could generate a lot of different ideas and give suggestions for what the family might try or what have helped other families we have previously met. Martin Söderquist also highlights the benefits of a reflection. The reflection should be based on what the family has said so far in the session and the language they have used. The therapist should also be free to add something. In a session with a couple that wanted to use "pause" when they argue at home, Söderquist brought this theme up in a reflection and suggested that the couple could use a "pause button". This was based on the goal the couple agreed on, but opened up a conversation on how to use such a *button*. Karen Story describes that after a reflection, the therapist should ask the couple or family for their feedback on the reflection. We should do this to create even more ways of talking about the subject. In Söderquist's case, the mentioning of a pause button is an example of an idea, originally coming from the couple, but where the therapist enlightens it further or brings new ideas into the discussion. Söderquist also emphasizes that we do not know what we create before or afterwards. This is just like golden moments, we cannot plan on when and how they will happen, but we can use the SST framework to detect new perspectives, discoveries and golden moments for the families we meet.

Summaries and the Takeaway

One of the clinical experiences that are in the foreground in trying to create significant moments is the use of summaries and takeaways. When talking to the five therapists it is clear that this is a part of SST that many see as important in offering a difference to the families they meet. Karen Story and Lynda Moore describe the process of a written summary for those who attend the session. If one is working in a team, a third or second therapist who is listening to the session can be the one to create such a summary. The goal is to listen for nuances of difference and new information that surfaces during the session. The therapist should listen for ways that we can make a difference for the family and what is happening relationally between them. The summary should carefully focus on what would be the most helpful for the family to have when they walk away. At the Bouverie Centre the summary is given to the family after the session and also stored at the clinic. This is done in case a family comes back and meets with a different therapist. A summary is described as something very post-modern, narrative and driven by the language of the family. It is not an assessment, nor diagnostic. Story says that "we use the words the family uses and we read it to them at the end of the session to ensure it is accurate, to ensure they feel understood and to allow the family to alter it if they want to". Tsorlinis adds that families often find it validating to hear themselves in the summary. It is a powerful part of the single session. Moore shares that "when we e-mail the summary, some answer back". One family wrote back that the summary had been an important part of the session, and something that they would read again and digested later on. "It's hard for families to remember things from sessions, so it's useful to have it written down so clients can review the session which can help them to be able to move forward", Tsorlinis describes. We can understand that the use of summaries, both in and after a session, is a way of offering reflections, giving something back to families, making them feel heard and remembering key parts of a session.

After a summary in a session and coming towards an ending, it might be useful to ask families for takeaways: "what are you bringing with you from this session or what is on your mind?" The takeaways will be included in the summary that is sent to the family. Jeff Young underlines the importance and significance of families having something to take away. He remembers a family he worked with that kept the "take away cards" from the sessions on their bedside table. They did so for their own motivation and for being reminded of what they had worked on in sessions. The part of a session creating the takeaways is often intense and reflects a cooperation between everyone in the room. A goal is that everyone in a family shares something they can take with them from the session, Moore says. This is then a way for therapists to understand and listen for significant or golden moments of a session. What has been useful to the family, what is not mentioned?

Being the Therapist

As a therapist, we never know what kind of themes, families, couples or challenges we will meet. In SST "You don't know what you are going to walk into or what will walk into you", Story says. There are different families every time and in SST there is a truly not-knowing way of working as it often does not require referral. Clients might simply walk-in. Using a team in sessions might help the collaborative process in the session. The possibility of working with teams varies greatly, and might not be possible where you, the reader, work. If possible, a team might be helpful in the summary process and makes it possible to debrief and do supervision after sessions.

One of the perspectives in SST is the idea that we might not meet again for more sessions. This could make therapists more courageous and address more of what comes to the surface in the conversation. It is important to ethically reflect on what we address and what we let by, as we need to make choices as to what to deal with in the limited time. As therapists it might also be difficult to balance alliance with the different individuals of a family. Story says that people often want the therapist to take sides, but we address it and say, "We will not do that". She experiences that people value the straightforwardness, and that it seems more inspiring for families to cut to the chase than spending energy on getting the therapist on their side.

When We Need More Than One Session or a Different Therapist

The relation between a therapist and a family, couple or other clients needs a certain chemistry, play and flow. It is hard to put into words what these words mean and how they look in practice, but Martin Söderquist describes that small misunderstandings in the communication makes it harder to get a proper flow in therapy, both in general and in SST. He once saw a mother and her daughter for therapy and was watching them as they played with toys and puppets by themself. He noticed a flow between the two as they played and noticed a link between the mother-daughter relationship and the relationship in a therapy room between the therapist and the family. "If it isn't a playful and dynamic conversation it will stop", Söderquist describes. At times it is not possible to be on the same frequency or understanding each other in the way it is intended.

This does not mean that there is something wrong with the therapist, or the client, as this is a relational challenge. This happens at times, and Söderquist recommends that therapists should be aware of this and end therapy or refer to someone else, if that is the best for the client.

Conclusion

There are many approaches and ways of working within systemic psychotherapy with couples and families. There are many ways therapists can contribute to change or significant moments in therapy. SST is a therapeutic frame available for both younger and more experienced therapists. As described, SST may be useful as a way of working in itself, or could simply be used as inspiration for making the most out of the *here and now* and the power, and strength of every session we have. It is important that therapists focus on the needs of those we meet and adapt style, amount of sessions and approach to help clients in the best possible way. I hope you have found this chapter inspiring for your own practice and that you might use the clinical experiences presented to reflect on your own practice: How are you spending the time with those you meet, what do you see as important steps in the therapeutic process and how do you create a space for significance in a session?

References

Andersen, S. R. (2021). Når en samtale er alt vi har [When one session is all we have]. I L. Lorås & J. C. V. Christensen (Red.), *Samtaler i relasjonelt arbeid* [Dialogues in relational work] (s. 231–246). Fagbokforlaget.

Bloom, B. (2001). Focused Single-Session Psychotherapy: A Review of the Clinical and Research Literature. *Brief Treatment and Crisis Intervention, 1*, 75–86.

Campbell, A. (2012). Single-session approaches to therapy: Time to review. *The Australian and New Zealand Journal of Family Therapy, 33*(1), 15–26. https://doi.org/10.1017/aft.2012.3

Doorn, K. A.-v., & Sweeney, K. (2019). The effectiveness of initial therapy contact: A systematic review. *Clinical Psychology Review, 74,* 1–14. https://doi.org/10.1016/j.cpr.2019.101786

Dryden, W. (2019). *Single-session therapy.* Routledge. https://doi.org/10.4324/9780429024313

Hoyt, M., Bobele, M., Slive, A., Young, J., & Talmon, M. (2018). *Single-session therapy by walk-in or appointment.* Routledge. https://doi.org/10.4324/9781351112437

Hoyt, M., Young, J., & Rycroft, P. (2020). Single session thinking 2020. *The Australian and New Zealand Journal of Family Therapy, 41*(3), 218–230. https://doi.org/10.1002/anzf.1427

Le Gros, J., Wyder, M., & Brunelli, V. (2019). Single session work: Implementing brief intervention as routine practice in an acute care mental health assessment service. *Australasian Psychiatry, 27*(1), 21–24. https://doi.org/10.1177/1039856218815756

O'Neill, I. (2017). What's in a name? Clients' experiences of single session therapy. *Journal of Family Therapy, 39*(1), 63–79. https://doi.org/10.1111/1467-6427.12099

Rose, S., Bisson, J. I., & Wessely, S. (2003). A systematic review of single-session psychological interventions ('debriefing') following trauma. *Psychotherapy and Psychosomatics, 72*(4), 176–184. https://doi.org/10.1159/000070781

Söderquist, M. (2020). *Ett samtal i taget. Familjerådgivning i ny form* [One session at a time. A new kind of family counselling]. Studentlitteratur.

Söderquist, M. (2023). *Single session one at a time counselling with couples. Challenge and possibility.* Routledge.

Talmon, M. (1990). *Single session solutions. A guide to practical, effective and affordable therapy.* Addison-Wesley.

Young, J., & Rycroft, P. (2012). Single session therapy: What's in a name? *The Australian and New Zealand Journal of Family Therapy, 33*(1), 3–5. https://doi.org/10.1017/aft.2012.1

Young, J., & Rycroft, P. (2020). *Single session thinking, self-paced online training suite.* The Bouverie Centre, La Trobe University.

11

Coming Full Circle with the Neuroscience: Using New Theory to Re-understand Therapy

Arlene Vetere

It is my contention in this chapter that all relational therapists and practitioners, whether working with individuals, couples, family systems, groups and teams, would benefit from a working knowledge of human anatomy and physiology. As systemic therapists we see relational suffering and as therapists we see people suffering—we work within and between relational experiences and their personal and contextual embeddedness. But, for too long has the body, and embodied experience, been sidelined within the systemic field of practice (Dallos & Vetere, 2022). It was not always so—the early family therapists worked directly with the body in therapeutic process and included an understanding of emotional and embodied experiences in their systemic formulations and interventions, and in the development of the therapeutic relationship, for example, Virginia Satir, Salvador Minuchin, Carl Whittaker, Murray Bowen and Chloe Madanes, amongst others (Vetere & Dallos, 2003). The

A. Vetere (✉)
VID Specialized University, Oslo, Norway

subsequent and so-called turn to narrative seemed to emphasise the significance of cognition and narration, but perhaps without always articulating how we learn to narrate, as children and young people, and what happens to the development of narrative ability in conditions of chronic fear and unhelpful arousal, for example. So, whilst it is very important to understand our cognitive and communicative processes, our narrative abilities and the impact of wider social and cultural factors on well-being and development, we may inadvertently live out a mind-body split in our understandings of distress and relational dilemmas and how we might be of assistance unless in addition we specifically theorise emotion, relational danger and bodily responses.

This chapter is not about a neuroscientific 'truth' but rather explores how human physiology and brain connectivity (integration) underpins our therapeutic relational work. I hope to show how some aspects of what therapists knew intuitively are borne out in relevant and recent neuroscience and, in doing so, draw on the work of researchers such as Alan Schore, Dan Siegel, Bessel van der Kolk, Pat Ogden, Judith Herman and Pat Crittenden. Thus these are the main concepts we shall be working with in the chapter: polyvagal theory; arousal regulation; autonomic nervous systems; fight-flight responding; relational danger; attachment and trauma; brain hemisphere functioning; and dispositional representations of experience.

The fragmenting of experience that we so often see in the face of relational trauma is physiological, psychological, interpersonal and cultural. We need relationships for our survival so exposure to unprotected and uncomforted relational dangers can impair the bonds of attachment security. For example, dissociation as a self-protective strategy makes danger and dangerous people less personal, or real. More extreme forms of defensive exclusion or dissociation can leave people feeling disconnected from self and others, with perhaps no safe havens or secure base (Bowlby, 1988). The effects of relational danger can feel deadening and our therapeutic task is to assist people to restore, repair and ground themselves without being overwhelmed in the process and by the process. Thus the safety of the therapeutic relationship is essential in promoting the conditions for trust, curiosity, learning and growth to thrive. Gottman's (2011) research suggests that accessibility, responsiveness and engagement are the building blocks of interpersonal trust in therapy. Thus we shall look at what we do, think, sense and feel in how we communicate empathy and co-regulate arousal in our therapeutic work.

In our work with children, adolescents and families we need to be able to draw on the emerging research on brain development, for example, sleep rhythms, the links between physical puberty and brain development, reward processing and the impact of childhood relational trauma on adolescent brain development. As systemic practitioners we need to translate this research into practice in a variety of life contexts and work settings for young people and their parents—helping with understanding that they are not alone in having complicated feelings (hormone imbalances, pruning), and that things will change with maturation—that their current experience is part of a process that moves them towards adulthood—with an increasing capacity for abstract thought, improvements in working memory and communication skills and scientific reasoning—the neuroscience helps us understand why adolescents are drowsy in the morning (melatonin still in the brain at this time), do not always understand consequences and how they can be assisted with motivation (role of dopamine/and importance of reward) and learning (arousal) (Blakemore, 2019).

Polyvagal theory (Porges, 2011) is now being used in the understanding and treatment of trauma. The theory describes and explains different states of the nervous system, for example, the concept of safety and social engagement means we need to work with clients in this state rather than when they are in a state of danger. This understanding links with our therapeutic observations and our experiences of working together in the room. Interoception is described as how we physiologically, and with conscious awareness, regulate the body signals that accompany our emotions. For example, it is possible to brain scan two people at once, to see how their brains respond to each other—in moments of emotional connection, their bodies, including their brains, actually physically synchronise. Thus this chapter is not about a neuroscientific 'truth'—it is more about how the experience of the psychotherapist with all their various theoretical knowledges can integrate with modern attachment theory and the science of arousal regulation, that is, how the different fields of study can inform each other. This profoundly challenges the conceptual split between mind and body. There have been many advances in our understanding of arousal, co-regulation and brain connectivity but they do not always easily translate into practices of healing. The Boston Change Process Study Group (2010) write about arousal regulation as a key to recovery in 'moments of meeting'. Following the earlier work of Watzlawick et al. (1974), change is seen as occurring in the small unremarkable moments as well as in the larger moments of discovery, founded in the properties of relationships. The Boston Group assert that the therapeutic relationship is a sufficient condition for therapeutic change. It is relationships that make the difference—as Bowlby observed, and as Dan Siegel says, we are all hardwired for connection!

Complex Trauma

Complex trauma responses in family members are more likely to develop with chronic exposure to relational danger, both visible and invisible dangers. Complex trauma responses are less responsive to traditional therapies because of factors like the severity and duration of the danger, the inter-generational nature of the danger, the developmental ages of children and the level and quality of social and emotional support available to parents and children. Stabilisation and emotional grounding is always the first stage in trauma-informed work with constant attention paid to the somatic aspects of trauma experiences. Some family members may never stabilise sufficiently to undertake more focused and demanding trauma therapy, such that the relational focus remains key, with an emphasis on support and a strengthening for what is going well.

We start together in relational therapy where people feel at their safest. We need to understand family members' preferred self-protective strategies and strategic positioning when they feel threatened, insecure and unsafe, such as a dismissing or arousal deactivating response strategy on the one hand, or on the other hand, a preoccupied and hyper-aroused response strategy with accompanying difficulty in down-regulating. This is where, and how, we meet them, that is, validating and supporting emotion and feeling with a more preoccupied response style, and validating and supporting cognition with a more dismissing response style. Therapy can be threatening and the implicit demand to develop a trusting relationship with a kindly stranger may be overwhelming.

In the face of relational danger, when we fear loss, rejection and/or abandonment, our fight-flight responses are activated. They are protective and healthy and designed to promote survival, but in the case of unresolved trauma and loss, they may be unhelpfully maintained by the body's continuing attempt to resolve the trauma responses (Levine, 2015). Levine writes that trying to 'complete' the unfinished situation of 'fight/flight' by rehearsing and ruminating simply embeds the neural pathways and leads to chronic stress. We need reduced stress as a precondition for new neural pathways to grow with new experiences of felt safety, in trusting therapy relationships and/or safe relationships within our communities. Neurological development is recognised to be relational, as we access, attune and receive the help and support of others. We understand also that new neural growth is supported by our conscious attention, that is, where we direct our attention, again with the assistance of trusted others, blood flow increases, which supports neuronal firing in ways that promote integration between disparate parts of the brain. The physiological response in fight-flight can be changes in heart rate, respiration, muscle tone, digestion, blood circulation, a state of alert and the release of stress neurochemicals such as adrenaline and cortisol. They may not be understood, monitored or managed by the person experiencing them. Intense emotions, such as fear, are stored as visceral sensations and felt as anxiety and panic and/or stored as visual images, such as flashbacks and nightmares. Flashbacks activate the right hemisphere of the brain and deactivate the left hemisphere. Even when we can talk about the danger, our body holds onto the physical manifestation of the event(s). Consequently and crucially, our body can be experienced as the cause of our distress rather than the dangerous events we have lived through. If the relational dangers occurred before language development or without the help of a safe adult to assist with making meaning of the events, reminders or 'triggers', such as sounds, smells, touch and sights, can lead to the continued release of stress hormones, the build-up of muscle tension and so on, which can result in later physical health problems (Levine, 2015; Ogden, 2021). The work of van der Kolk (2014) was crucial in pointing the way to working somatically to heal the trauma, as well as psychologically and relationally. The psychological impact of danger can be expressed as changes in the biological stress response and a psychological loss of who we are, and relationally as a loss of secure connection.

Healing the body is supported by the neuroscience with its developing understanding of how frightening and shameful experiences can be disconnected within the brain, for example, and how some of these processes are not under explicit voluntary control—'can't, not won't' as Dan Siegel (2009) puts it! However, we do not translate these neuroscientific understandings directly into therapeutic techniques. As systemic therapists we see relational suffering and as therapists we see people suffering—we work within and between relational experiences and their personal and contextual embeddedness. Our therapeutic task is often to help bring to conscious (left brain) awareness that which is held implicitly in relational procedural and sensory memory, so that we might then 'walk around' in these warded off experiences, with the help and support of the therapist and in the safety of the therapeutic relationship. This can take many forms in relational therapy—direct work, witnessing work, coaching and support, indirect work and so on. The neuroscience informs us as we explore experiences of felt safety in connection, and experiences of joy and transcendence, to recognise unresolved loss and hurt in relationships, to understand the impact of emotional neglect and chronic fear, to recognise the significance of comfort and reassurance in relationships, and how we have learned to protect ourselves and others. Experiences of not being loved, listened to, believed and taken seriously can reduce our sense of agency and personal power. It can become harder to have a clear sense of who we are when our self-regulation is not supported relationally.

Dispositional Representations

Exposure to developmentally normal dangers and learning to comfort and protect, both self and others, is a part of our resilient responding. When we are comforted and protected in these ways we learn that we can trust others. However some dangers are inflicted by parents, or the events/ relationships are also dangerous to the parent, and/or the dangers are chronic. In these circumstances, the absence of comfort and protection for the child can lead to adaptive distortions in their thinking and responding that can either exaggerate or minimise the probability of relational danger. And when there is no safe adult to help the child make sense of dangerous events, the child does their best to predict future danger and organise their own protective responses. Attachment theory attempts to help us understand how, and under what interpersonal conditions, our self-protective strategies develop, and similarly how they can be revised in the light of new information (Crittenden, 2008).

Damasio (1999) suggests that our attachment representations are dispositional; that is, we are predisposed to respond in difficult interpersonal moments based on the environment/relational context and our remembered experiences of past responding. Our dispositional representations are thought to be neurological patterns of activity resulting from all our interactions, including our thoughts, with our attachment figures. Our representations are tied to our memory systems and are organised according to somatic, cognitive or affective information, and in terms of whether they are preverbal or potentially verbal memories. They are reworked each time we think of an attachment figure.

For example, Jane and her partner, Steve, sought therapy because every time they tried to have sexual intercourse, Jane was overcome by her 'throat anxiety' as she called it. Her throat would close and she would fear she was suffocating. As a loving couple this caused them both distress as they struggled to understand the nature of this difficulty. In the therapy, with the help of her own cognition, Jane connected her 'throat anxiety' to earlier sexual abuse from her grandfather. However, cognition does not always over-ride somatic/sensory memory, especially when grounded in fear of early danger, so the therapeutic 'space' offered the opportunity to slowly and gently illuminate and expand understanding, for both of them.

Integration and Self-Reflexivity

Schore and Schore (2008) write of the potential for the brain's right hemisphere involvement in therapeutic work, especially when addressing relational trauma. Our more cognitive left hemisphere understandings, explorations and verbal responses to interpretation may not be sufficient for family members to feel stable enough to face the challenges of addressing frightening or shameful trauma memories. Our task is to recruit both right and left brain hemispheres' memory resources through action, and vision, for example, alongside cognition and verbal competence. The systemic therapies have developed many action-based interventions that can help recruit our right and left brain memory resources, for example, emotional sculpting with coins and small objects, internalised other interviewing, attachment-oriented genograms, systemic tracking of both difficult and successful interpersonal moments and experiences, empty chair work, visual scaling questions, externalising problematic relational cycles, family drawings and tree of life work. Working with vision and colour, with drawings, for example, and with action helps to activate the memory resources of the right brain. We are helping to bring to conscious awareness that which is held implicitly in memory. Similarly, systemic interventions can be adapted to assist family members with 'warming up' when dismissing or minimising emotional information has been protective, that is, exploring warded off aspects of experience and taking the risk of naming and addressing difficult emotional responses. The energy needed for this can be considerable and need not be underestimated. We assist with 'calming down', that is, developing strategies to cope with overwhelming feelings, to calm, comfort and soothe, both self and other, when this has not been available or possible in the past. If people live with hyper-aroused states, we assist by working slowly, perhaps using systemic tracking methods, to pause and to reflect to allow the needed time for processing. We all need to be sufficiently calm to think about what is happening, and what our responses might be during difficult interpersonal moments to avoid harmful or hurtful interpersonal escalations. When we cross the threshold into fight/flight responding, with concomitant physiological flooding, it may be that our only option for self-regulation is quiet recovery time and some breathing space, literally. And as we calm down, and our reflective capacity is once again engaged, we can see our other options. If we are working with family member(s) who employ more extreme dismissing responses in difficult interpersonal moments, as therapists we may not always be aware of their need to breathe and calm themselves. Within a systemic framework, with our focus on process and 'talking about talking' we may be able to predict some of these moments and agree how we proceed. Neurofeedback training is increasingly recommended by psychotherapists of most schools for these reasons, along with promoting understanding of how our brains and bodies work during both difficult moments and safer ones; learning the comfort and soothing of self-compassion and developing a belief we are entitled to such care; learning to turn to others for understanding and help with emotional regulation; and weaving these understandings within our faith and spirituality. Bodily based therapies, using dance, yoga, movement and theatre are being developed to support emotional regulation and the processing of implicit memory. Van der Kolk (2014) concludes that all therapies aim to assist the process of self-observation as the only currently known pathway that we have to reorganise the perceptual systems of the brain.

We know that the physical/emotional presence of someone we trust can reduce or quell our fear response in the face of a relational threat or danger. This person acts as a powerful safety signal. Erica Hornstein et al. (2022), at UCLA, published an article in the journal *Emotion*, suggesting that physical warmth can do the same thing, that is, naturally inhibit our fear responding. We know that 'bear hugs' stimulate the release of oxytocin, and endogenous opioids—and warmth—it seems, can also affect our fear learning. Are these similar neural pathways perhaps implicated in mammalian survival?

The Advent of Polyvagal Theory

For years, psychotherapists have worked with extreme states of anxiety and depression and have understood the role of the autonomic nervous system (ANS) in regulating states of arousal. Polyvagal theory (Porges, 2011) has finessed our understanding of the ANS cycle of engagement, mobilisation and disconnection. Engagement (ventral vagal parasympathetic) is considered to be a calm state, where social co-operation is optimal. Mobilisation is our fight/flight (sympathetic) response state. In the face of danger, the vagal 'brake' is disengaged, and the sympathetic system takes over as adrenaline and cortisol are released. Our ability to read facial cues is affected and we may see 'neutral' faces as angry or dangerous faces; our information-processing capacity slows down; and we become preoccupied with our own affective state. In the face of extreme danger, the dorsal vagal system takes over. Disconnection is the dorsal vagal parasympathetic state of 'freeze'. Our parasympathetic system has two branches—dorsal and ventral vagal. Ventral vagal is our parasympathetic 'brake', regulating arousal, maintaining optimum arousal and returning to a safe state. Dorsal vagal shuts down digestion and slows breathing and heart rate in extreme states of fear.

Our ANS responds to the everyday challenges in our lives, letting us know how we are, not who or what we are. Neuroception, or sub-cortical detection without conscious awareness, manages risks and dangers by changing our physiological state. Usually the shifts are subtle, but in the face of a single event danger, for example, our ANS needs to be sufficiently resilient to return to a regulated state. As we discussed earlier, the sympathetic system manages the arousal needed for fight/flight responding. Our survival and well-being rely on our ability to down-regulate our states of defence with states of safety and trust. This explains why a reassuring smile or a hug can be so soothing and calming for us. However, exposure to constant danger can explain why our neural reactions can be reset towards a defensive bias and how they lose resilience to return to a state of safety. Although this is adaptive behaviour in the face of constant danger, it can help explain why people who hold unprocessed trauma responses find it harder to engage with others as the ANS process of building safe connections has been interrupted. For example, when a child was exposed to danger without comfort, protection or assisted with meaning-making, they constructed their best explanation of what happened with their existing cognitive resources at the time and a rule to stay safe. This rule (or strategy) was designed to protect at that time, but becomes increasingly mis-attuned to circumstances and maladaptive over time. If the child developed a more preoccupied strategy they are increasingly likely to over-estimate the probability of danger, as an automatic procedural response, and a more dismissing strategy suggests the likely forgetting of the event(s) that no one talks about (Crittenden & Heller, 2017). Dan Siegel suggests that unresolved trauma shows as states of chaos or as states of rigidity, and the more stressed a system becomes (person and/or group), the more likely we are to see these polarising processes. Therapy is designed to help us move to integration and to more states of flexibility, where our growing sense of safety and security helps us adapt, reflect, organise our thoughts and feelings, and live embodied and relational lives, where we regulate the flow of energy and information, neither constantly underwhelmed nor overwhelmed, and thus linking our differentiated parts of experience.

Deb Dana (2018) sees therapy through a polyvagal lens as a process of assisting family members to re-pattern the ways their ANS operates when the drive to survive competes with the longing to connect with others. So, just as the brain can change, so can the ANS be intentionally influenced. For example, she advocates assisting people to identify their autonomic states, to track their response patterns in different interpersonal situations, to recognise their triggers for arousal (questioning: what is the danger? …or, is it a past resonance?), to identify and practise their regulatory resources so that they might increase the regulating capacity of their ventral vagal system. Dana emphasises the significance of co-regulation, that is, reciprocal regulation of autonomic states with trusted others, mediated by our mirror neurons, so that we begin to feel safe enough to connect and enter into other trusting relationships. If we live in relationships characterised by hurt and mis-attunement, we orient to danger and survival, but if we are supported by co-regulating relationships we become resilient. We are not only assisting with self-regulation in therapy, but with the freedom that allows the body to relax because it is met with empathy and care. As therapists we may at times need to be reminded to relax and to play in the therapeutic process for the sake of loving relations and freedom.

Here we can see a direct connection with Bowlby's work on the attachment system as a learned response to safety and danger, and Crittenden's later research on the development of self-protective strategies and the impact of living with 'dismissed' trauma. For example, an unhelpful escalation between a couple can also be seen as the communication of danger signals between two nervous systems that triggers the need for protection. The ANS is not seen to make judgements about good or bad responses, but rather learned protective responses, often below the level of conscious awareness. Appreciating the protective intent of our ANS responses can help reduce experiences of shame and blame in couple/family therapy. Here the attunement of the therapist can assist initially with signals of safety and an invitation for connection such that compassion and our brain's pre-frontal capacity for curiosity can be activated. Van der Kolk suggests that in these circumstances of danger we need to understand that perception is more important than reality—it is the perception of an experience that creates trauma responses, and polyvagal theory helps explain that even before the brain makes meaning, the ANS has assessed the environment for danger and initiated an adaptive survival response. Thus neuroception is seen to precede perception. Story follows state. The question 'Are you interested in exploring what just happened here?' perhaps following a family member's momentary dissociation, is designed to explore the autonomic response and thus facilitate conscious processing, that is, helping to link thoughts with somatic experience. Similarly, a therapeutic request to 'notice that', followed by the question 'what happens next?', can assist in being curious about cues of safety and danger. This can facilitate a family or couple in navigating the path towards a greater sense of relational safety. Re-storying, as a therapeutic process, is thus underpinned by awareness of our autonomic states, recognition of our adaptive survival responses and our increased capacity to regulate and co-regulate into a ventral vagal state.

Polyvagal theory suggests that through the social engagement system we both send and seek cues of safety. Dana writes about a therapeutic process of pendulation, whereby family members are intentionally helped to move between states of activation and calm—thus experimenting with the safe release of the vagal brake and re-engagement of the brake. This is similar to Minuchin's (1974) emphasis on enactment as a therapeutic process, and its deployment by Johnson (2018) in emotionally focused couple and family therapy. We see here the ANS underpinning of the titration of lived experience, with pacing, timing and parsing of experience. In more extreme situations of dissociation, flat affect and inactivation, she writes of the therapist's 'gentle call to action' to reactivate sympathetic energy. As Crittenden writes, cognition cannot always override procedural/sensory memory, so this emphasis on bringing to conscious awareness a realisation of our own ANS state and that of our loved ones, in difficult moments, both remembered and actual, begins the process of over-ride, or reaching the body. This can be seen as one of the biggest challenges in therapy for both therapists and clients—as clients may say, 'I understand what is happening but my body does not stop reacting and takes control of me'.

'Don't ask what's wrong with me. Ask what's happened to me'.

Suzanne O'Sullivan (2021) writes of psychosomatic problems or functional neurological disorders, as they are now called—real physical symptoms that are disabling, and which are understood to have a psychological or behavioural cause. Currently, treatments are either physical or psychological, and cut across any integrated bio-psycho-social understanding and thus do not avoid the mind-body split with the provision of separate treatment pathways. She critiques the need for us as practitioners to join our socio-political and cultural languages with that of the biology of behaviour. In her work, she has spoken to many people across different communities and come to understand how the richness of people's stories can shape their expressions of distress. She tries also to frame their experiences in biological terms to give substance to the physiological reality of their conditions. The social contributions to psychosomatic problems are harder for individual practitioners to address, risking an inward look that could lead to the individual feeling blamed for their condition—whereas a systemic approach always seeks to recruit resources, especially those of social and spiritual support in the community: family, friends, work/educational colleagues, faith leaders and so on. Perhaps we sometimes need to be reminded of the possibility to invite others who have healing potential, such as friends and relatives, and include them directly in the therapeutic work.

We see a systemic example in the stress-system model of Kasia Koslowska and her colleagues (2020) whereby attachment relationships, adverse childhood experiences and neurobiology interact within a family community context of overwhelming demands. Children can suffer disturbances of neuro-physiological regulation and Koslowska et al. write sensitively and at length as to how to communicate this to distressed families and children. Symptomatic behaviour or presenting problems, as they are called, can have a functional meaning in the context of past exposure to relational danger with a link to the present time. This might involve exploring past experiences of comfort, or its lack, the self-protective function of symptomatic behaviour, and/or unhelpful transformations of information, all of which were in the service of adaptation and survival, for example, what is the missing information—thought or feeling? What was the past experience of danger and how was it processed? How did your body help you to survive?

We embody the narrative and that reciprocally influences how we tell the story. Our attachment experiences shape, and in turn, are re-shaped by our narratives—how we are able to develop and construct stories—what is forgotten, minimised, dismissed, celebrated, exaggerated, integrated and reflected upon. Thus what we are able to narrate, in turn shapes our attachment patterns. We are meaning-making people and we rely on coherence to communicate clearly and straightforwardly so that others might grasp the fullness of our experiences. Whereas our trauma responses of flashbacks, interrogation, rumination, intrusions and hypervigilance—these are elements of a scattered life narrative trying to put itself back together. Bowlby understood that we are always seeking connection and integration, even though we might not know what it looks like, feels like and how to do it. Repetition of the experience of safety, perhaps initially with the help and support of a therapist or predictable other person, helps us to restore coherence and our commitment to our own well-being.

Conclusion

The recent neuroscientific research helps us understand how an integrated state of mind brings us into a more mindful, reflective and embodied sense of what is happening in the here and now, both personally and relationally. We are able to use our curiosity to differentiate experiences in the present moment. The responsibility for us as therapists is to develop our capacity for self-regulation in the face of distress, our own, and that of others, whereby we can deconstruct our own subjective responses (Wampold, 2011). This helps us stay compassionate and attuned, with 'right brain' to 'right brain' communication, asking, 'What just happened there?' (Schore & Schore, 2008). If someone, ourselves and/or family members are physiologically flooded they cannot readily tolerate complexity, and we need to restrain ourselves from adding complexity to the narrative at this time—the richer account, as it is called. We need to attend to preferred self-protective strategies as this is how we hold complexity. We try to be in a relationship with another's mental state, to enter a process of interactive regulation. We have a process orientation in our systemic therapies. We are trained to observe process: our own, that of our clients and our growing mutuality. Thus the reflective practitioner develops their understanding of their own attachment strategies in the face of others' unhelpful physiological arousal, and the conditions under which their own strategies are activated and engaged. Learning to regulate our arousal and to co-regulate with others is seen as a key self-function on which other functions can develop, such that we can stay present, open and focused with the extremes that we all experience, such as grief, sadness, rage and anger. A systemic supervision process is so helpful for us as therapists to find ways to be calmer and to support family members to repair and heal their relationships in ways to aid the reorganisation of their experiences (Vetere & Sheehan, 2017).

Psychiatric diagnoses remain uncertain descriptions of symptomatic behaviour. Psychiatric medications may help with symptomatic suffering but do not address the main causes of human suffering, for example, the lack of acknowledgement of past heartbreak, loss, shame and fear. We work in therapy towards coherence and a sense of an integrated self, for our clients, our supervisees and ourselves: to be someone who can name and articulate their own distress, and who can connect up their thoughts, feelings, actions and intentions, and observe them, in dialogue with someone who listens, sees and understands.

References

Blakemore, S. J. (2019). Adolescence and mental health. *The Lancet, 393*(10185), 2030–2031. https://doi.org/10.1016/S0140-6736(19)31013-X

Boston Change Process Study Group. (2010). *Change in psychotherapy: A unifying paradigm*. Norton.

Bowlby, J. (1988). *A secure base*. Basic Books.

Crittenden, C., & Heller, M. (2017). The roots of chronic post-traumatic stress disorder: childhood trauma, information processing and self-protective strategies. *Chronic Stress (Thousand Oaks)*. https://doi.org/10.1177/24705 47016682965

Crittenden, P. (2008). *Raising parents: Attachment, parenting and child safety.* Willan Publishers.

Dallos, R., & Vetere, A. (2022). *Systemic therapy and attachment narratives* (2nd ed.). Routledge.

Damasio, A. (1999). *The feeling of what happens: Body, emotion and the making of consciousness.* Heinemann.

Dana, D. (2018). *The polyvagal theory in therapy: Engaging the rhythm of regulation.* Norton.

Gottman, J. (2011). *The science of trust: Emotional attunement for couples.* Norton.

Hornstein, A., Fanselow, M., & Eisenberger, N. (2022). Warm hands, warm hearts: An investigation of physical warmth as a prepared safety stimulus. *Emotion, 22*(7), 1517–1528. https://doi.org/10.1037/emo0000925

Johnson, S. (2018). *Attachment theory in practice: Emotionally focused therapy with individuals, couples and families.* Guilford Press.

Koslowska, K., Scher, S., & Helgeland, H. (2020). *Functional somatic symptoms in children and adolescents.* Palgrave Macmillan.

Levine, P. (2015). *Trauma and memory: Brain and body in a search for the living past.* North Atlantic Books.

Minuchin, S. (1974). *Families and family therapy.* Harvard University Press.

O'Sullivan, S. (2021). *The sleeping beauties and other stories of mystery illness.* Pan Macmillan.

Ogden, P. (2021). *The pocket guide to sensorimotor psychotherapy in context.* Norton.

Porges, S. W. (2011). *The polyvagal theory: Neurophysioological foundations of emotions, attachment, communication and self-regulation.* Norton.

Schore, A., & Schore, J. (2008). Modern attachment theory: The central role of affect regulation in development and treatment. *Clinical Social Work Journal, 36*, 9–20.

Siegel, D. (2009). *Mindsight: The new science of personal transformation.* Bantam.

Van der Kolk, B. (2014). *The body keeps the score: Brain, mind and body in the healing of trauma.* Penguin Random House.

Vetere, A., & Dallos, R. (2003). *Working systemically with families.* Karnac.

Vetere, A., & Sheehan, J. (Eds.). (2017). *Supervision of family therapy and systemic practice.* Springer.

Wampold, B. (2011). *Qualities and actions of effective therapists. Continuing education in psychology.* American Psychological Association.

Watzlawick, P., Weakland, J., & Fisch, R. (1974). *Change: Principles of problem formation and problem resolution.* Norton.

12

Epilogue

Tone Grøver, Siv Merete Myra, and Ulf Axberg

When we started working on this book, many countries in the world were still in lockdown because of the Covid pandemic, including the countries of the authors. Lockdowns had lasted for almost two years, and our daily lives had gone through changes we could not have imagined before the pandemic. We developed new vocabularies and new ways of relating. And we experienced a clear feeling of how unpredictable and vulnerable life is. At the same time there are so many other uncertainties, like the effects of climate changes, destabilization of democracies, uncertain economic futures for many, migration, refugee flows and wars. We clearly feel how dependent we are on each other, as well as how difficult this interdependence can be.

T. Grøver (✉) • S. M. Myra • U. Axberg
Department of Family Therapy and Systemic Practice, Faculty of Social Studies, VID Specialized University, Oslo, Norway
e-mail: Tone.Grover@vid.no; siv.merete.myra@vid.no; ulf.axberg@vid.no

T. Grover et al. (eds.), *New Horizons in Systemic Practice with Adults*, Palgrave Texts in Counselling and Psychotherapy, https://doi.org/10.1007/978-3-031-30526-9_12

In times of uncertainty like these, we wondered if, and how, this could affect our systemic thinking, and our systemic ways of working together with families, couples and individuals who seek to relate to their lives together with us. It would have been understandable if we sought more security, simplifications and something clearer and firmer to hold on to in the systemic field.

Without knowing how the authors would relate to the uncertainty and the pressure we are surrounded with, we asked them to write about what occupies them now, in relation to their own practice. As the chapters came back to us, we could clearly see that what inspires the authors in their different contexts is not at all something firmer and simpler. On the contrary, we saw existential themes as the most striking in the chapters. The authors are concerned with getting close to the micro-systems in the relationships they are involved in, in their work, at the same time as they ask big philosophical and existential questions, turning around the complexity of what they see and encounter. And it is questions, not answers, that dominate. We see them turn their questions around themes of love, trust, spirituality, loneliness and community, creativity, identity, the significance of poetry, longing and questions around forgiveness. We see authors dare to open the questions, without approaching answers or conclusions. We see that the authors have confidence in the reader: What will be important for the reader in the development of their own practices? Can this book inspire you to come closer to your own questions?

Therefore, this book is a part of a process, in our common desire to keep the systemic field in motion. We started the book with a chapter recognizing Love, understood as Agape, in therapy, and it ends with "coming full circle". Even though we ask questions, and are taking not-knowing positions, there is something we know: all the latest research on human neurobiology confirms what we have held as a guideline in systemic therapy—the quality of the relationship, in its most fragile, subtle and playful forms. In such a way, we are glad we could include understandings from poetry to neuroscience, from experiences of lived lives to philosophy, from spirituality to learning from ecosystems. And maybe this bridging to many disciplines is an important part in the future development of the systemic era?

If we are to make any "conclusions" about the essence of the chapters perhaps it goes like this: We should keep our hearts warm, our sensitivity at the highest, our humility for those we meet in our work contexts and the knowledge they have about themselves and their lives, as our most important values in a systemic understanding. And not least in times of uncertainty. Ethics seems to be more important than techniques or methods, for all the authors.

What do you think will be most important for you, dear reader?

Index[1]

---

[1] Note: Page numbers followed by 'n' refer to notes.

© The Author(s), under exclusive license to Springer Nature Switzerland AG 2023   **183**
T. Grover et al. (eds.), *New Horizons in Systemic Practice with Adults*, Palgrave Texts in
Counselling and Psychotherapy, https://doi.org/10.1007/978-3-031-30526-9

The manufacturer's authorised representative in the EU is Springer
Nature Customer Service Centre GmbH, Europaplatz 3, 69115 Heidelberg,
Germany. If you have any concerns regarding our products, please
contact ProductSafety@springernature.com

Printed and bound by CPI Group (UK) Ltd, Croydon, CR0 4YY
06/05/2026
02104301-0001